The No-Diet PCOS FERTILITY Food List & Meal Plan

Balance Your Hormones, Regulate Your Cycle, and Boost Ovulation in 30 Days — Without The Sad & Bland Foods

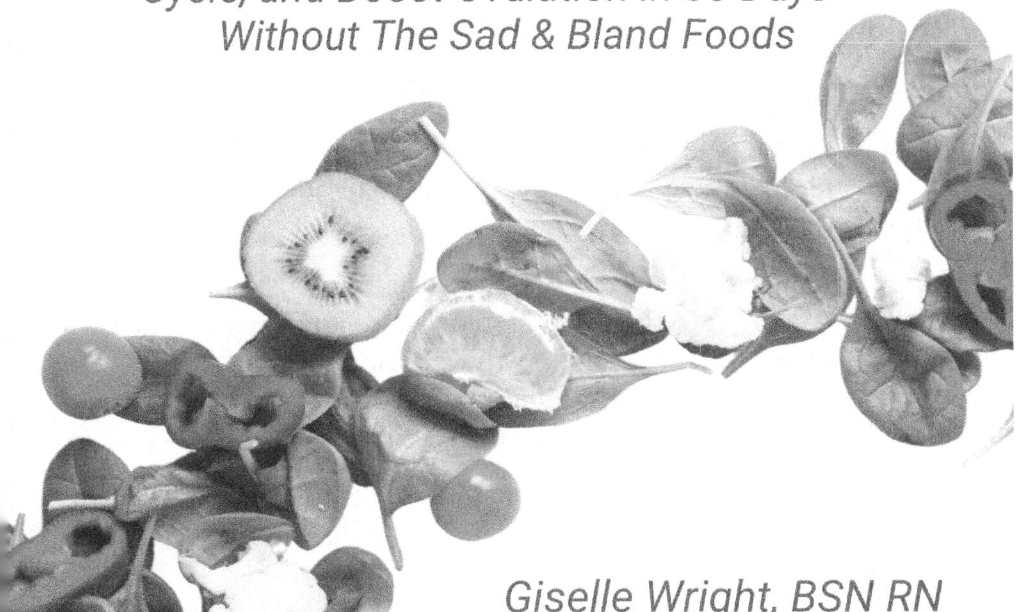

Giselle Wright, BSN RN
PCOS Nurse Expert

Giselle Wright, BSN RN
Binnovate Publishers

Dedication

To the women who are in this same battle. You have been an encouragement to me to keep moving forward and to keep on searching for answers. It blesses me to know that I am not alone in this, and makes me positive that we can win this, in whatever shape or form victory may come.

To John, my beloved husband. You have been my solid rock. Cooking with and for me, taking me for a random beach drive so I can diffuse and destress, prepping my bike so we can go on quick rides despite our busy schedules. Oh! Having you in my life is truly a gift. I love you. <3

Other books by Giselle Wright, BSN RN on Amazon!

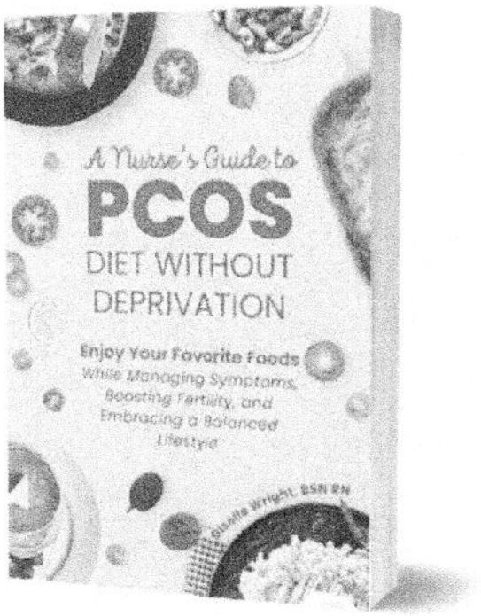

Nurse's Guide to PCOS Diet Without Deprivation: Enjoy Your Favorite Foods While Managing Symptoms, Boosting Fertility, and Embracing a Balanced Lifestyle

https://www.amazon.com/dp/1966232306

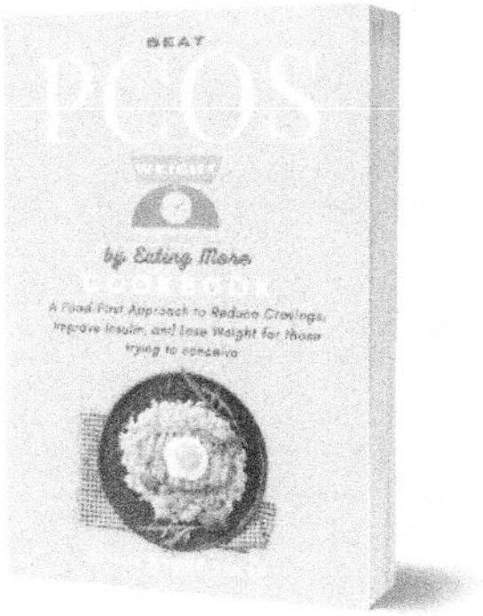

Beat PCOS Weight By Eating More Cookbook: A Food-First Approach to Reduce Cravings, Improve Insulin, and Lose Weight for those trying to conceive

https://www.amazon.com/dp/1966232330

Table of Contents

Introduction: Understanding PCOS and Fertility

Polycystic Ovary Syndrome (PCOS) is a prevalent hormonal disorder that affects approximately 1 in 10 women of reproductive age. This condition is characterized by a combination of symptoms, including irregular menstrual cycles, elevated androgen levels, and the presence of polycystic ovaries. For many women, PCOS can lead to a range of challenges, particularly concerning fertility.

Women with PCOS often experience irregular ovulation or anovulation, which can complicate the journey to conception. The hormonal imbalances associated with PCOS disrupt the delicate interplay of hormones necessary for ovulation and pregnancy. Understanding these dynamics is crucial for women seeking to manage their symptoms and improve their reproductive health.

While the diagnosis of PCOS can feel overwhelming, it is essential to recognize that effective management strategies exist. By gaining knowledge about the condition and its effects on fertility, women can take proactive steps toward enhancing their chances of conception and overall well-being.

The Importance of Nutrition in Managing PCOS

Nutrition is a cornerstone of effective PCOS management and plays a vital role in enhancing fertility. Research has shown that dietary choices can significantly influence insulin sensitivity, hormone balance, and overall health. Many women with PCOS experience insulin resistance, which can lead to weight gain and exacerbate symptoms.

Adopting a balanced diet focused on whole, nutrient-dense foods can stabilize blood sugar levels, reduce inflammation, and support hormonal balance. This book emphasizes the importance of nutrition as a foundational element in managing PCOS and improving fertility outcomes.

Incorporating specific foods known to support hormonal health empowers women to take charge of their fertility journey. The right dietary choices can lead to improved energy levels, mood stabilization, and even modest weight loss, all of which can enhance the chances of conception.

Overview of the Book's Structure

"The No-Diet PCOS Fertility Food List & Meal Plan" is designed to provide practical, science-backed guidance for women with PCOS who are trying to conceive. The book is structured to offer clear, actionable information, making it easy for readers to implement dietary changes into their daily lives.

Chapter 1: The Science of PCOS and Insulin Resistance

How Insulin Resistance Affects Fertility

Insulin resistance is a hallmark of Polycystic Ovary Syndrome (PCOS) and plays a significant role in the condition's symptoms and complications. In a healthy body, insulin helps regulate blood sugar levels by facilitating the uptake of glucose into cells for energy. However, in individuals with insulin resistance, the body's cells become less responsive to insulin, leading to elevated blood sugar levels.

This condition can trigger a cascade of hormonal imbalances, particularly affecting the ovaries. Elevated insulin levels can increase the production of androgens (male hormones) such as testosterone, which can disrupt the normal ovulatory process. High androgen levels can lead to irregular menstrual cycles, anovulation, and other symptoms associated with PCOS, such as acne and excessive hair growth.

Moreover, insulin resistance can contribute to weight gain, which further exacerbates hormonal imbalances. Studies have shown that even a modest weight loss of 5-10% can significantly improve insulin sensitivity, restore regular ovulation, and enhance fertility outcomes for women with PCOS. Therefore, addressing insulin resistance is crucial for managing PCOS and improving reproductive health.

The Role of Blood Sugar Balance in PCOS Management

Maintaining blood sugar balance is essential for women with PCOS, as it directly impacts insulin sensitivity and overall hormonal health. A diet that stabilizes blood sugar levels can help mitigate the effects of insulin resistance and support fertility.

Key Strategies for Blood Sugar Balance:

Choose Low Glycemic Index (GI) Foods: Foods with a low glycemic index release glucose slowly into the bloodstream, preventing spikes in blood sugar and insulin levels. Examples include whole grains, legumes, non-starchy vegetables, and most fruits. Incorporating these foods into meals can help maintain steady energy levels and reduce cravings.

Prioritize Protein and Healthy Fats: Including adequate protein and healthy fats in meals can enhance satiety and slow down the absorption of carbohydrates. This combination helps stabilize blood sugar levels and reduces the likelihood of insulin spikes. Consider incorporating sources like lean meats, fish, eggs, nuts, seeds, and avocados into your diet.

Regular Meal Timing: Eating at regular intervals can help prevent drastic fluctuations in blood sugar levels. Aim for three balanced meals and healthy snacks throughout the day to keep energy levels stable and support metabolic health.

Stay Hydrated: Drinking plenty of water is essential for overall health and can aid in maintaining blood sugar balance. Sometimes, feelings of hunger can be mistaken for thirst, so staying hydrated can help manage cravings.

Incorporate Physical Activity: Regular exercise can improve insulin sensitivity and help manage weight. Aim for a combination of aerobic activities (like walking, cycling, or swimming) and strength training to support overall health and hormonal balance.

Understanding PCOS: Metabolic Reproductive Syndrome

An alternative name for Polycystic Ovary Syndrome is Metabolic Reproductive Syndrome. This term emphasizes the metabolic aspects of the condition, highlighting that PCOS is not solely about the presence of cysts in the ovaries. In fact, the so-called "cysts" are actually immature follicles that have not developed properly due to hormonal imbalances.

Why the Alternative Name Matters

Broader Understanding: Referring to PCOS as Metabolic Reproductive Syndrome helps shift the focus from just the reproductive symptoms to the metabolic issues that are often present, such as insulin resistance, obesity, and dyslipidemia.

Holistic Approach: This name encourages a more holistic approach to treatment, addressing both metabolic and reproductive health. It underscores the importance of lifestyle changes, including diet and exercise, in managing the condition.

Reducing Stigma: By moving away from the term "polycystic," which can lead to misconceptions about the condition being solely about ovarian cysts, the alternative name helps reduce stigma and promotes a better understanding of the multifaceted nature of PCOS.

Understanding PCOS as Metabolic Reproductive Syndrome can empower women to take a more comprehensive approach to their health, focusing on both metabolic and reproductive aspects of the condition.

Chapter 2: Top 10 Fertility-Boosting Foods

Incorporating specific foods into your diet can significantly enhance fertility and support hormonal balance, especially for women with PCOS. Here are ten fertility-boosting foods, along with their benefits, macronutrient profiles, and practical tips for including them in your meals.

1. Avocados

Why They Help: Avocados are rich in healthy monounsaturated fats, which support hormone production and help maintain stable blood sugar levels. They are also packed with folate, a vital nutrient for reproductive health.

Macros (per 1 medium avocado):

- *Calories: 240*

- *Protein: 3g*
- *Carbohydrates: 12g*
- *Fat: 22g*

How to Incorporate: Enjoy 1/4 to 1/2 an avocado daily. Add it to smoothies, spread it on whole-grain toast, or use it as a creamy base for salad dressings. You can also make guacamole for a delicious dip with veggies or whole-grain chips.

2. Leafy Greens (Spinach, Kale)

Why They Help: Leafy greens are high in folate, iron, and magnesium, all essential for ovulation and early pregnancy. They also provide antioxidants that combat oxidative stress, which can negatively impact fertility.

Macros (per 1 cup raw spinach):

- *Calories: 7*
- *Protein: 1g*
- *Carbohydrates: 1g*
- *Fat: 0g*

How to Incorporate: Add a handful of spinach or kale to your morning smoothie, toss them into omelets, or sauté them with garlic and olive oil as a side dish. Consider making a hearty salad with mixed greens, nuts, and a light vinaigrette.

3. Berries

Why They Help: Berries, such as blueberries, strawberries, and raspberries, are rich in antioxidants and fiber. They help reduce inflammation and oxidative stress in the ovaries, while their natural sweetness can satisfy sugar cravings without spiking blood sugar.

Macros (per 1 cup mixed berries):

- *Calories: 70*
- *Protein: 1g*
- *Carbohydrates: 17g*
- *Fat: 0g*

How to Incorporate: Use berries as a go-to sweet snack or dessert. Top yogurt or oatmeal with fresh berries, blend them into smoothies, or enjoy them frozen as a refreshing treat.

4. Fatty Fish (Salmon, Sardines)

Why They Help: Fatty fish are loaded with omega-3 fatty acids, which reduce inflammation and may improve egg quality. Omega-3s also support healthy cervical mucus and a balanced mood, both important for fertility.

Macros (per 3 oz cooked salmon):

- *Calories: 206*
- *Protein: 22g*
- *Carbohydrates: 0g*
- *Fat: 13g*

How to Incorporate: Aim for 2-3 servings of fatty fish per week. Grill or bake salmon, add sardines to salads or pasta dishes, or try making fish tacos with avocado and cabbage slaw. If you're not a fish fan, consider plant-based omega-3 sources like walnuts and chia seeds.

5. Citrus Fruits (Oranges, Lemons)

Why They Help: Citrus fruits are natural sources of myo-inositol, a compound shown to improve insulin sensitivity and ovulation in women with PCOS. They are also rich in vitamin C, which supports overall health and immune function.

Macros (per 1 medium orange):

- *Calories: 62*
- *Protein: 1g*
- *Carbohydrates: 15g*
- *Fat: 0g*

How to Incorporate: Squeeze lemon juice into your water for a refreshing drink, enjoy an orange as a midday snack, or add slices of grapefruit to your breakfast. You can also use citrus zest to enhance the flavor of baked goods and dressings.

6. Nuts and Seeds (Walnuts, Flaxseeds)

Why They Help: Nuts and seeds are excellent sources of healthy fats, protein, and essential nutrients like vitamin E and magnesium. They support hormone production and can help reduce inflammation.

Macros (per 1 oz walnuts):

- *Calories: 185*
- *Protein: 4g*
- *Carbohydrates: 4g*
- *Fat: 18g*

How to Incorporate: Snack on a handful of mixed nuts, sprinkle flaxseeds on your morning oatmeal or yogurt, or blend them into smoothies. Consider making energy balls with nuts, seeds, and dried fruit for a nutritious on-the-go snack.

7. Whole Grains (Quinoa, Brown Rice)

Why They Help: Whole grains are rich in fiber, which helps regulate blood sugar levels and supports digestive health. They also provide essential nutrients like B vitamins, which are important for energy metabolism and hormone regulation.

Macros (per 1 cup cooked quinoa):

- *Calories: 222*
- *Protein: 8g*
- *Carbohydrates: 39g*
- *Fat: 4g*

How to Incorporate: Use quinoa or brown rice as a base for salads, stir-fries, or grain bowls. Swap out white rice and pasta for whole grain alternatives, and experiment with different grains like farro or barley for variety.

8. Legumes (Chickpeas, Lentils)

Why They Help: Legumes are high in protein and fiber, making them excellent for stabilizing blood sugar levels. They also provide essential nutrients like iron and folate, which are important for reproductive health.

Macros (per 1 cup cooked lentils):

- *Calories: 230*
- *Protein: 18g*
- *Carbohydrates: 40g*
- *Fat: 1g*

How to Incorporate: Add chickpeas to salads, blend them into hummus, or use lentils in soups and stews. Consider making a lentil salad with diced vegetables and a light dressing for a nutritious meal.

9. Sweet Potatoes

Why They Help: Sweet potatoes are a great source of complex carbohydrates, fiber, and beta-carotene, which the body converts to vitamin A. This nutrient is essential for hormone production and reproductive health.

Macros (per 1 medium sweet potato):

- *Calories: 112*
- *Protein: 2g*
- *Carbohydrates: 26g*
- *Fat: 0g*

How to Incorporate: Roast sweet potatoes as a side dish, mash them with a little olive oil and seasoning, or use them in soups and stews. You can also slice them thinly and bake them for a healthy chip alternative.

10. Greek Yogurt

Why They Help: Greek yogurt is rich in protein and probiotics, which support gut health and hormone balance. The calcium and vitamin D in yogurt are also important for reproductive health.

Macros (per 1 cup plain Greek yogurt):

- *Calories: 100*
- *Protein: 17g*
- *Carbohydrates: 6g*
- *Fat: 0g*

How to Incorporate: Enjoy Greek yogurt as a snack or breakfast topped with berries and nuts. Use it as a base for smoothies, or incorporate it into salad dressings and sauces for added creaminess.

Incorporating these fertility-boosting foods into your diet can help support hormonal balance and enhance your chances of conception. Remember, small changes can lead to significant improvements in your overall health and well-being.

While this chapter is fairly helpful, I have prepared a more comprehensive chart of foods that you can eat and avoid or limit in chapter 4. Making this book a handy tool you can carry along with you in the grocery store or just about anywhere where food is involved.

Chapter 3: The Power of Whole Foods

In the journey toward managing PCOS and enhancing fertility, the quality of the foods you consume plays a crucial role. Whole foods, which are minimally processed and close to their natural state, offer numerous health benefits compared to their processed counterparts. This chapter explores the advantages of whole foods, how to read labels effectively, and tips for making informed dietary choices.

Benefits of Whole Foods vs. Processed Foods

Whole Foods

Whole foods include fruits, vegetables, whole grains, nuts, seeds, legumes, and unprocessed meats and dairy. These foods are typically rich in essential nutrients, including vitamins, minerals, fiber, and antioxidants. Here are some key benefits of incorporating whole foods into your diet:

- ***Nutrient Density:*** Whole foods are packed with nutrients that support overall health and hormonal balance. They provide essential vitamins and minerals that are often lacking in processed foods.

- ***Fiber-Rich***: Whole foods are generally high in dietary fiber, which aids digestion, helps regulate blood sugar levels, and promotes satiety. Fiber is particularly important for women with PCOS, as it can help manage insulin resistance.

- ***Lower in Added Sugars and Unhealthy Fats***: Whole foods typically contain fewer added sugars and unhealthy fats compared to processed foods. This can help stabilize blood sugar levels and reduce inflammation, both of which are crucial for managing PCOS.

- ***Natural Antioxidants***: Many whole foods are rich in antioxidants, which help combat oxidative stress and inflammation in the body. This is particularly beneficial for women with PCOS, as inflammation can exacerbate symptoms.

Processed Foods

Processed foods, on the other hand, are often high in added sugars, unhealthy fats, and sodium, while being low in essential nutrients. Examples include sugary snacks, fast food, and pre-packaged meals. Here are some drawbacks of consuming processed foods:

- ***Nutrient Deficiency***: Processed foods often lack the vitamins and minerals found in whole foods, leading to potential nutrient deficiencies over time.

- ***Blood Sugar Spikes***: Many processed foods have a high glycemic index, which can cause rapid spikes in blood sugar and insulin levels. This can worsen insulin resistance and contribute to weight gain.

- ***Additives and Preservatives***: Processed foods often contain artificial additives, preservatives, and flavor enhancers that can negatively impact health. Some of these substances may disrupt hormonal balance and contribute to inflammation.
- ***Increased Cravings***: The high sugar and fat content in processed foods can lead to cravings and overeating, making it challenging to maintain a healthy diet.

How to Read Labels and Make Informed Choices

Understanding food labels is essential for making informed dietary choices. Here are some tips for reading labels effectively:

- ***Check the Ingredients List***: The ingredients list is typically arranged in descending order by weight. Look for whole food ingredients at the top of the list. If you see a long list of unfamiliar additives or preservatives, it's a sign that the product is highly processed.
- ***Look for Whole Grains***: When choosing grain products, look for terms like "whole grain" or "whole wheat" as the first ingredient. Avoid products that list refined grains, such as "white flour," as the primary ingredient.
- ***Watch for Added Sugars***: Be mindful of added sugars, which can appear under various names (e.g., sucrose, high fructose corn syrup, agave nectar). Aim to choose products with little to no added sugars.
- ***Pay Attention to Serving Sizes***: Serving sizes can be misleading. Always check the serving size to understand the nutritional content accurately. A product may seem low in calories, but if the serving size is small, you may consume more than you realize.
- ***Consider Nutritional Content***: Look for products that are high in fiber, protein, and healthy fats while being

low in saturated fats, trans fats, and sodium. Aim for foods that provide a good balance of macronutrients.

- ***Be Cautious with Health Claims***: Many processed foods make health claims (e.g., "low-fat," "sugar-free") that can be misleading. Always read the ingredients and nutritional information to determine if the product aligns with your health goals.

By prioritizing whole foods and learning to read labels effectively, you can make informed choices that support your health and fertility. This approach not only helps manage PCOS symptoms but also fosters a sustainable and enjoyable way of eating.

Chapter 4: The Ultimate PCOS Food List

Managing Polycystic Ovary Syndrome (PCOS) involves making informed dietary choices that support hormonal balance and overall health. This chapter provides a comprehensive food list categorized by food groups, highlighting foods to include and limit, along with their nutritional information.

How to Use the Charts

Navigating the food list is simple! Here's a step-by-step guide to help you utilize the charts effectively:

1. Categorization: The charts are organized into general food groups:

   Fruits, Vegetables, Proteins, some Grains for Carbs, and Healthy Fats.

2. Standardized Measurements: Each food group is further categorized by preparation styles, standardized to a measurement of 100 grams. Below this, you will find

additional measurements (slices, teaspoons, tablespoons, pieces, serving, oz, or cups) along with their corresponding weights in grams.

3. Nutrient Information: For each 100 grams of food, you will find the corresponding amounts of essential nutrients, including:

    - Calories
    - Carbohydrates
    - Proteins
    - Fats
    - Sodium
    - Phosphorus
    - Potassium

4. Calculating Nutrient Content: You can divide or multiply the nutrient values based on the amount of food you are preparing in your recipe.

Example 1: Actual Nutrient Content in Your Recipe

Asparagus	Serving Quantity	Serving Unit	Calories (kCal)	Protein (g)	Total Carbohydrates (g)	Sodium (mg)	Potassium (mg)	Phosphorus (mg)	Total Fat (g)
boiled, drained	100.0	g	22	2.4	4.1	14.00	224.0	54.00	0.22
	90.00	g	20	2.2	3.7	12.60	201.6	48.60	0.20
	0.50	c							

Let's say your recipe calls for 1 cup of boiled asparagus. According to the food list chart, 90 grams of boiled asparagus is equivalent to ½ cup. Since you need a full cup, you would multiply the nutrient values by 2.

For 1 cup of asparagus, the nutrient content would be:

- Calories: 40 kCal
- Protein: 4.4 g
- Carbohydrates: 7.4 g
- Fats: 0.40 g
- Sodium: 25.2 mg
- Potassium: 403 mg

- Phosphorus: 97.2 mg

Example 2: More on Reading and Using the Chart

Asparagus	SERVING QUANTITY	SERVING UNIT	CALORIES (kcal)	PROTEIN (g)	TOTAL CARBOHYDRATES (g)	SODIUM (mg)	POTASSIUM (mg)	PHOSPHORUS (mg)	TOTAL FAT (g)
boiled, drained	100.0	g	22	2.4	4.1	14.00	224.0	54.00	0.22
	90.00	g	20	2.2	3.7	12.60	201.6	48.60	0.20
	0.50	c							
frozen	100.0	g	24	3.2	4.1	8.00	253.0	64.00	0.23
	87.00	g	21	2.8	3.6	6.96	220.1	55.68	0.20
	6.00	pcs							

Consider 6 pieces of frozen asparagus, which weigh approximately 87 grams. You would reference the nutrient values based on the 87-gram line. If you wish to reduce your total carbohydrates intake, you might choose to eat only 3 pieces, which would lower the carbs content from 3.6 g to approximately 1.8g.

Alternatively, using a kitchen scale to measure your food allows you to adjust your intake based on the 100-gram standard, tailoring your consumption to meet your daily needs and restrictions effectively.

Frails

Apple

	SERVING QUANTITY	SERVING UNIT	CALORIES (kCal)	PROTEIN (g)	TOTAL CARBOHYDRATES (g)	SODIUM (mg)	POTASSIUM (mg)	PHOSPHORUS (mg)	TOTAL FAT (g)
Gala, raw, with skin	100.00	g	57	0.3	13.7	1.00	108.00	11.00	0.12
	172.00	g	98	0.4	23.5	1.72	185.76	18.92	0.21
	1.00	pc, med							
fuji, raw,with skin	100.00	g	63	0.2	15.2	1.00	109.00	13.00	0.18
	192.00	g	121	0.4	29.2	1.92	209.28	24.96	0.35
	1.00	pc, med							
golden delicious, with skin	100.00	g	57	0.3	13.6	2.00	100.00	10.00	0.15
	169.00	g	96	0.5	23.0	3.38	169.00	16.90	0.25
	1.00	pc, med							
granny smith, w/ skin, raw	100.00	g	58	0.4	13.6	1.00	120.00	12.00	0.19
	167.00	g	97	0.7	22.7	1.67	200.40	20.04	0.32
	1.00	pc, med							
juice, frozen concentrate	100.00	g	47	0.1	11.5	7.00	126.00	7.00	0.10
	239.00	g	112	0.3	27.6	16.73	301.14	16.73	0.24
	8.00	fl oz							
applesauce, sweetened, canned	100.00	g	68	0.2	17.5	2.00	75.00	6.00	0.17
	123.00	g	84	0.2	21.5	2.46	92.25	7.38	0.21
	0.50	c							
applesauce, unsweetened, canned	100.00	g	42	0.2	11.3	2.00	74.00	5.00	0.10
	122.00	g	51	0.2	13.8	2.44	90.28	6.10	0.12
	0.50	c							

Blackberries

raw	100.00	g	43	1.4	9.6	1.00	162.00	22.00	0.49
	144.00	g	62	2.0	13.8	1.44	233.28	31.68	0.71
	1.00	c							
frozen, unsweetened	100.00	g	64	1.2	15.7	1.00	140.00	30.00	0.43
	151.00	g	97	1.8	23.7	1.51	211.40	45.30	0.65
	1.00	c							
canned, heavy syrup	100.00	g	92	1.3	23.1	3.00	99.00	14.00	0.14
	256.00	g	236	3.4	59.1	7.68	253.44	35.84	0.36
	1.00	c							

Raspberries

raw	100.00	g	52	1.2	11.9	1.00	151.00	29.00	0.69
	123.00	g	64	1.5	14.7	1.23	185.73	35.67	0.80
	1.00	c							
frozen, unsweetened	100.00	g	56	1.2	12.6	4.00	184.00	30.00	0.81
	140.00	g	78	1.6	17.6	5.60	257.60	42.00	1.13
	1.00	c							
red, frozen, sweetened, unthawed	100.00	g	103	0.7	26.2	1.00	114.00	17.00	0.16
	125.00	g	129	0.9	32.7	1.25	142.50	21.25	0.20
	0.50	c							
puree, w/ seeds. Juice concentrate	100.00	g	55	na	11.5	4.00	195.00	30.00	0.97
	100.00	G	221	3.0	53.2	10.00	1,178	100	1.34

Blueberries	SERVING QUANTITY	SERVING UNIT	CALORIES (kCal)	PROTEIN (g)	TOTAL CARBOHYDRATES (g)	SODIUM (mg)	POTASSIUM (mg)	PHOSPHORUS (mg)	TOTAL FAT (g)
fresh	100.00	g	57	0.7	14.5	1.00	77.00	12.00	0.33
	145.00	g	83	1.1	21.0	1.45	111.65	17.40	0.48
	1.00	c							
sweetened, dried	100.00	g	317	2.5	80.0	3.00	214	36.00	2.50
	40.00	g	127	1.0	32.0	1.20	85.60	14.40	1.00
	0.25	c							
wild, frozen	100.00	g	57	0.0	13.9	3.00	68.00	13.00	0.16
	140.00	g	80	0.0	19.4	4.20	95.20	18.20	0.22
	1.00	c							
unsweetened, frozen	100.00	g	51	0.4	12.2	1.00	54.00	11.00	0.64
	155.00	g	79	0.7	18.9	1.55	83.70	17.05	0.99
	1.00	c							
canned, light syrup , drained	100.00	g	88	1.0	22.7	3.00	54.00	12.00	0.40
	244.00	g	215	2.5	55.3	7.32	131.76	29.28	0.98
	1.00	c							

Strawberries

Strawberries	SERVING QUANTITY	SERVING UNIT	CALORIES (kCal)	PROTEIN (g)	TOTAL CARBOHYDRATES (g)	SODIUM (mg)	POTASSIUM (mg)	PHOSPHORUS (mg)	TOTAL FAT (g)
fresh, whole	100.00	g	32	0.7	7.7	1.00	153	24.00	0.30
	144.00	g	46	1.0	11.1	1.44	220.3	34.56	0.43
	1.00	c							
unsweetened, frozen (unthawed)	100.00	g	35	0.4	9.1	2.00	148	13.00	0.11
	149.00	g	52	0.6	13.6	2.98	220.5	19.37	0.16
	1.00	c							
sweetened, frozen, thawed	100.00	g	78	0.5	21.0	1.00	98.00	12.00	0.14
	127.50	g	99	0.7	26.8	1.28	124.9	15.30	0.18
	0.50	c							
fruit topping	100.00	g	254	0.2	66.3	21	51.00	5.00	0.10
	42.00	g	107	0.1	27.9	8.82	21.42	2.10	0.04
	2.00	tbsp							
pastry, 23pprox, enriched	100.00	g	371	5.4	47.8	445	83.00	89.00	18.50
	71.00	g	263	3.8	33.9	316	58.93	63.19	13.14
	1.00	pc							
Milkshake (fastfood)	100.00	g	113	3.4	18.9	83	182	100	2.80
	226.40	g	256	7.7	42.8	188	412	226.4	6.34
	8.00	fl oz							
yogurt, low fat 1 item = 1 container	100.00	g	105	8.2	12.3	33.0	129.0	109.0	2.57
	150.00	g	158	12	18.4	49.5	193.5	163.5	3.86
	1.00	item							

Cherries	SERVING QUANTITY	SERVING UNIT	CALORIES (kCal)	PROTEIN (g)	TOTAL CARBOHYDRATES (g)	SODIUM (mg)	POTASSIUM (mg)	PHOSPHORUS (mg)	TOTAL FAT (g)
sweet, without pits	100.00	g	63	1.1	16.0	0.00	222.00	21.00	0.20
	154.00	g	97	1.6	24.7	0.00	341.88	32.34	0.31
	1.00	c							
sour red, without pits	100.00	g	50	1.0	12.2	3.00	173.00	15.00	0.30
	155.00	g	78	1.6	18.9	4.65	268.15	23.25	0.47
	1.00	c							
juice, tart	100.00	g	59	0.3	13.7	4.00	161.00	17.00	0.54
	269.00	g	159	0.8	36.9	10.76	433.09	45.73	1.45
	1.00	c							
Pitanga or Surinam	100.00	g	33	0.8	7.5	3.00	103.00	11.00	0.40
	173.00	g	57	1.4	13.0	5.19	178.19	19.03	0.69
	1.00	c							
tart, dried, sweetened	100.00	g	333	1.3	80.5	13.00	376.00	36.00	0.73
	40.00	g	133	0.5	32.2	5.20	150.40	14.40	0.29
	0.25	c							
maraschino, canned, drained	100.00	g	165	0.2	42.0	4.00	21.00	3.00	0.21
	5.00	g	8	0.0	2.1	0.20	1.05	0.15	0.01
	1.00	pc/ item							
sweet, canned in juice, pitted	100.00	g	54	0.9	13.8	3.00	131.00	22.00	0.02
	250.00	g	135	2.3	34.5	7.50	327.50	55.00	0.05
	1.00	c							
sweet, canned in water	100.00	g	46	0.8	11.8	1.00	131.00	15.00	0.13
	248.00	g	114	1.9	29.2	2.48	324.88	37.20	0.32
	1.00	c							
sweet, frozen, sweetened thawed	100.00	g	89	1.2	22.4	1.00	199.00	16.00	0.13
	259.00	g	231	3.0	57.9	2.59	515.41	41.44	0.34
	1.00	c							
pie filling, canned 1/8 of 21 oz can = 1 svg	100.00	g	115	0.4	28.0	18.00	105.00	15.00	0.07
	74.00	g	85	0.3	20.7	13.32	77.70	11.10	0.05
	1.00	svg							
pie fillings, low calorie	100.00	g	53	0.8	12.0	12.00	118.00	15.00	0.16
	264.00	g	140	2.2	31.6	31.68	311.52	39.60	0.42
	1.00	c							
sour red, canned in water, drained	100.00	g	42	0.7	10.5	4.00	115.00	16.00	0.21
	168.00	g	71	1.2	17.6	6.72	193.20	26.88	0.35
	1.00	c							
sour red, 24pprox.24ned, frozen unthawed	100.00	g	46	0.9	11.0	1.00	124.00	16.00	0.44
	155.00	g	71	1.4	17.1	1.55	192.20	24.80	0.68
	1.00	c							

Grapefruit	Serving Quantity	Serving Unit	Calories (kCal)	Protein (g)	Total Carbohydrates (g)	Sodium (mg)	Potassium (mg)	Phosphorus (mg)	Total Fat (g)
fresh	100.00	g	32	0.6	8.1	0.00	139.0	8.00	0.10
	153.33	g	49	1.0	12.4	0.00	213.13	12.27	0.15
	0.67	c							
white, fresh, small (3.5 diameter)	100.00	g	33	0.7	8.4	0.00	148.0	8.00	0.10
	118.00	g	39	0.8	9.9	0.00	174.6	9.44	0.12
	0.50	pc							
pink or red	100.00	g	42	0.8	10.7	0.00	135.0	18.00	0.14
	153.33	g	64	1.2	16.4	0.00	207.0	27.60	0.21
	0.67	c							
juice, white	100.00	g	39	0.5	9.2	1.00	162.0	15.00	0.10
	247.00	g	96	1.2	22.7	2.47	400.1	37.05	0.25
	8.00	fl oz							
juice, pink	100.00	g	39	0.5	9.2	1.00	162.0	15.00	0.10
	247.00	g	96	1.2	22.7	2.47	400.1	37.05	0.25
	1.00	c							
juice, unsweetened, pink, canned	100.00	g	37	0.6	7.5	2.00	141.0	17.00	0.66
	247.20	g	91	1.4	18.6	4.94	348.6	42.02	1.63
	8.00	fl oz							

Pears									
whole, medium (2.5/lb)	100.00	g	57	0.4	15.2	1.00	116.0	16.00	0.14
	166.00	g	95	0.6	25.3	1.66	192.6	19.92	0.23
	1.00	pc							
halves, canned in water	100.00	g	29	0.2	7.8	2.00	53.00	7.00	0.03
	244.00	g	71	0.5	19.1	4.88	129.3	17.08	0.07
	1.00	c							
Asian	100.00	g	42	0.5	10.7	0.00	121.0	11.00	0.23
	122.00	g	51	0.6	13.0	0.00	147.6	13.42	0.28
	1.00	pc							

Avocados									
fresh, raw mashed/ pureed	100.00	g	160	2.0	8.5	7.00	485	52.00	14.66
	230.00	g	368	4.6	19.6	16.10	1,120	120	33.70
	1.00	c							
California, raw/fresh no seed and skin	100.00	g	167	2.0	8.6	8.00	507.0	54.00	15.41
	136.00	g	227	2.7	11.8	10.9	690.0	73.40	21.00
	1.00	pc/ item							
Florida, fresh/ raw no seed and skin	100.00	g	120	2.2	7.8	2.00	351.0	40.00	10.06
	304.00	g	365	6.8	23.8	6.08	1,070	122.0	30.60
	1.00	pc/ item							
Guacamole	100.00	g	155	2.0	8.5	344	472.	51.00	14.18
	15.00	g	23	0.3	1.3	51.6	70.80	7.65	2.13
	1.00	tbsp							
oil	100.00	g	884	0.0	0.0	0.00	0.00	0.00	100
	14.00	g	124	0.0	0.0	0.00	0.00	0.00	14.00
	1.00	tbsp							

Lemon	SERVING QUANTITY	SERVING UNIT	CALORIES (kCal)	PROTEIN (g)	TOTAL CARBOHYDRATES (g)	SODIUM (mg)	POTASSIUM (mg)	PHOSPHORUS (mg)	TOTAL FAT (g)
whole,	100	g	20	1.2	10.7	3.00	145.0	15.00	0.30
without seeds	108	g	22	1.3	11.6	3.24	156.6	16.20	0.32
	1.00	pc/ item							
peeled, 2-	100	g	29	1.1	9.3	2.00	138.0	16.00	0.30
1/8" in	58.00	g	17	0.6	5.4	1.16	80.04	9.28	0.17
diameter)	1.00	pc/ item							
juice, fresh	100	g	22	0.4	6.9	1.00	103.0	8.00	0.24
	30.50	g	7	0.1	2.1	0.31	31.42	2.44	0.07
	1.00	fl oz							
peel or zest	100.0	g	47	1.5	16.0	6.00	160.0	12.00	0.30
	2.00	g	1	0.0	0.3	0.12	3.20	0.24	0.01
	1.00	tsp							
pudding mix	100.0	g	363	0.1	91.8	506.00	5.00	3.00	0.50
1 svg = ½ c	21.20	g	77	0.0	19.5	107.27	1.06	0.64	0.11
1 package = 85g	1.00	svg							
juice, canned	100.0	g	17	0.5	5.6	24.00	109.0	9.00	0.07
	30.50	g	5	0.1	1.7	7.32	33.25	2.75	0.02
	1.00	fl oz							
soda, lemon	100.0	g	40	0.1	24.9	9.00	1.00	0.00	0.02
lime	245.6	g	98	0.1	10.1	22.10	2.46	0.00	0.05
	8.00	fl oz							
juice,	100.0	g	22	0.5	6.5	1.00	89.00	8.00	0.32
unsweetened	5.08	g	1	0.0	0.3	0.05	4.52	0.41	0.02
, frozen	1.00	tsp							
pudding,	100.0	g	125	0.1	25.0	140.00	1.00	5.00	3.00
ready to eat	142.0	g	178	0.1	35.5	198.80	1.42	7.10	4.26
1 can= 5 oz	1.00	can/ item							
tea, black,	100.0	g	45	0.0	10.8	3.00	14.00	1.00	0.22
sweetened,	271.0	g	122	0.0	29.3	8.13	37.94	2.71	0.60
ready to drink	1.00	c							
Lime									
whole, 2" in	100.0	g	30	0.7	10.5	2.00	102.0	18.00	0.20
diameter	67.00	g	20	0.5	7.1	1.34	68.34	12.06	0.13
	1.00	pc/ item							
juice, fresh	100.0	g	25	0.4	8.4	2.00	117.0	14.00	0.07
	5.13	g	1	0.0	0.4	0.10	6.01	0.72	0.00
	1.00	tsp							
juice,	100.0	g	21	0.3	6.7	16.00	75.00	10.00	0.23
unsweetened	246.0	g	52	0.6	16.5	39.36	184.5	24.60	0.57
, canned	1.00	c							
frozen ice	100.0	g	128	0.4	32.6	22.00	3.00	1.00	0.00
dessert	99.00	g	127	0.4	32.3	21.78	2.97	0.99	0.00
	0.50	c							

Orange	SERVING QUANTITY	SERVING UNIT	CALORIES (kCal)	PROTEIN (g)	TOTAL CARBOHYDRATES (g)	SODIUM (mg)	POTASSIUM (mg)	PHOSPHORUS (mg)	TOTAL FAT (g)
whole, 2-5/8" diameter	100.00	g	47	0.9	11.8	0.00	181.0	14.00	0.12
	131.00	g	62	1.2	15.4	0.00	237.11	18.34	0.16
	1.00	pc/ item							
Valencia (California)	100.00	g	49	1.0	11.9	0.00	179.0	17.00	0.30
	135.00	g	66	1.4	16.1	0.00	241.6	22.95	0.41
	0.75	c							
Navel (California)	100.00	g	49	0.9	12.5	1.00	166.0	28.46	0.15
	123.75	g	61	1.1	15.5	1.24	205.4	23.00	0.19
	0.75	c							
Clementines	100.00	g	47	0.9	12.0	1.00	177.0	21.00	0.15
	74.00	g	35	0.6	8.9	0.74	131	15.54	0.11
	1.00	pc/ item							
orange sections	100.00	g	47	0.9	11.8	0.00	181.0	14.00	0.12
	135.00	g	63	1.3	15.9	0.00	244.4	18.90	0.16
	0.75	c							
juice	100.00	g	45	0.7	10.4	1.00	200.0	17.00	0.20
	248.00	g	112	1.7	25.8	2.48	496.0	42.16	0.50
	8.00	fl oz							
Florida, sections 1 fruit = 141g	100.00	g	46	0.7	11.5	0.00	169.0	12.00	0.21
	138.75	g	64	1.0	16.0	0.00	234.5	16.65	0.29
	0.75	c							
soda	100.00	g	48	0.0	12.3	12.0	2.00	1.00	0.00
	248.00	g	119	0.0	30.5	29.8	4.96	2.48	0.00
	8.00	fl oz							
marmalade	100.00	g	246	0.3	66.3	56.0	37.00	4.00	0.00
	20.00	g	49	0.1	13.3	11.20	7.40	0.80	0.00
	1.00	tbsp							
juice, frozen	100.00	g	95	0.5	23.2	8.00	100.0	13.00	0.00
	238.40	g	70	0.4	17.2	5.92	74.00	9.62	0.00
	1.00	c							
orange peel zest	100.00	g	97	1.5	25.0	3.00	212.0	21.00	0.20
	2.00	g	2	0.0	0.5	0.06	4.24	0.42	0.00
	1.00	tsp							
juice, unsweetened, canned	100.00	g	47	0.7	11.0	4.00	184.0	17.00	0.15
	249.00	g	117	1.7	27.4	9.96	458.2	42.33	0.37
	8.00	fl oz							
Mandarin, canned in juice	100.00	g	37	0.6	9.6	5.00	133.0	10.00	
	249.00	g	92	1.5	23.8	12.5	331.17	24.90	
	1.00	c							
juice, light, no pulp	100.00	g	21	0.2	5.4	4.00	188.0	4.00	
	240.00	g	50	0.5	13.0	9.60	451.2	9.60	
	8.00	fl oz							
Mandarin, canned in light syrup	100.00	g	61	0.5	16.2	6.00	78.00	10.00	
	252.00	g	154	1.1	40.8	15.12	196.6	25.20	
	1.00	c							

Foods to Limit

- Dried Fruits (Raisins, Dates)
    - Nutrition (per 1 oz raisins):
        - Calories: 85
        - Protein: 1g
        - Carbohydrates: 22g
        - Fat: 0g
    - Reason: High in sugar and calories, which can spike blood sugar levels.
- Fruit Juices
    - Nutrition (per 1 cup orange juice):
        - Calories: 112
        - Protein: 2g
        - Carbohydrates: 26g
        - Fat: 0g
    - Reason: Often high in sugar and low in fiber, leading to rapid blood sugar spikes.
- High Sugar Fruits
    - Banana, Grapes, Mangoes, and Pineapple
    - While these fruits contain natural sugars and will definitely create a blood sugar spike, they are also packed with beneficial fiber, vitamins, and antioxidants, so they can still be enjoyed but with caution and in moderation, especially when managing your insulin resistance and blood glucose levels.

Vegetables

Spinach

Spinach	SERVING QUANTITY	SERVING UNIT	CALORIES (kCal)	PROTEIN (g)	TOTAL CARBOHYDRATES (g)	SODIUM (mg)	POTASSIUM (mg)	PHOSPHORUS (mg)	TOTAL FAT (g)
raw, chopped	100.00	g	23	2.9	3.6	79.0	558.0	49.00	0.39
	90.00	g	21	2.6	3.3	71.10	502.2	44.10	0.35
	3.00	c							
frozen	100.00	g	29	3.6	4.2	74.0	346.0	49.00	0.57
	78.00	g	23	2.8	3.3	57.7	269.9	38.22	0.44
	0.50	c							
chopped, boiled, drained, no salt	100.00	g	23	3.0	3.8	70.0	466.0	56.00	0.26
	90.00	g	21	2.7	3.4	63.0	419.4	50.40	0.23
	0.50	c							

Swiss Chard

Swiss Chard	SERVING QUANTITY	SERVING UNIT	CALORIES (kCal)	PROTEIN (g)	TOTAL CARBOHYDRATES (g)	SODIUM (mg)	POTASSIUM (mg)	PHOSPHORUS (mg)	TOTAL FAT (g)
raw	100.00	g	19	1.8	3.7	213	379	46.00	0.20
	36.00	g	7	0.7	1.4	76.7	136.4	16.56	0.07
	1.00	c							
boiled, drained, no salt	100.00	g	20	1.9	4.1	179	549	33.00	0.08
	175.00	g	35	3.3	7.2	313	960.8	57.75	0.14
	1.00	c							

Arugula

Arugula	SERVING QUANTITY	SERVING UNIT	CALORIES (kCal)	PROTEIN (g)	TOTAL CARBOHYDRATES (g)	SODIUM (mg)	POTASSIUM (mg)	PHOSPHORUS (mg)	TOTAL FAT (g)
raw, leaves	100.00	g	25	2.6	3.7	27.0	369.0	52.00	0.66
	80.00	g	20	2.1	2.9	21.6	295.2	41.60	0.53
	4.00	c							
salad mixed baby greens Arugula butterhead, endives,Radicchio	100.00	g	18	1.5	3.3	16.9	298.7	32.15	0.27
	41.25	g	7	0.6	1.4	6.99	123.	13.26	0.11
	1.00	c							

Kale

Kale	SERVING QUANTITY	SERVING UNIT	CALORIES (kCal)	PROTEIN (g)	TOTAL CARBOHYDRATES (g)	SODIUM (mg)	POTASSIUM (mg)	PHOSPHORUS (mg)	TOTAL FAT (g)
raw, chopped	100.00	g	35	2.9	4.4	53.0	348.0	55.00	1.49
	83.75	g	29	2.5	3.7	44.4	291.5	46.06	1.25
	1.25	c							
chopped, boiled, drained, no salt	100.00	g	36	2.9	5.3	16.0	144.0	42.00	1.21
	65.00	g	23	1.9	3.5	10.4	93.60	27.30	0.79
	0.50	c							
scotch, raw, chopped	100.00	g	42	2.8	8.3	70.0	450.0	62.00	0.60
	83.75	g	35	2.4	7.0	58.6	376.9	51.93	0.50
	1.25	c							
scotch, boiled, drained, chopped no salt	100.00	g	28	1.9	5.6	45.0	274.0	38.00	0.41
	86.67	g	24	1.7	4.9	39.0	237.5	32.93	0.36
	0.67	c							
frozen, raw 1 pack=10 oz/ 284g	100.00	g	28	2.7	4.9	15.0	333.0	29.00	0.46
	85.05	g	24	2.3	4.2	12.76	283.2	24.66	0.39
	3.00	oz							
frozen, chopped, boiled, drained, no salt	100.00	g	36	2.9	5.3	16.0	144.0	42.00	1.21
	65.00	g	23	1.9	3.5	10.4	93.60	27.30	0.79
	0.50	c							

Broccoli	SERVING QUANTITY	SERVING UNIT	CALORIES (kCal)	PROTEIN (g)	TOTAL CARBOHYDRATES (g)	SODIUM (mg)	POTASSIUM (mg)	PHOSPHORUS (mg)	TOTAL FAT (g)
florets, raw	100.0	g	28	3.0	5.1	27.00	325.0	66.00	0.35
	71.00	g	20	2.1	3.6	19.17	230.7	46.86	0.25
	1.00	c							
Cooked, no salt	100.0	g	35	2.4	7.2	41.00	293.0	67.00	0.41
	78.00	g	27	1.9	5.6	31.98	228.5	52.26	0.32
	0.50	c							
frozen, spears	100.0	g	29	3.1	5.4	17.00	250.0	59.00	0.34
	85.05	g	25	2.6	4.6	14.46	212.6	50.18	0.29
	3.00	oz							

Cauliflower

green,raw	100.0	g	31	3.0	6.1	23.00	300.0	62.00	0.30
	64.00	g	20	1.9	3.9	14.72	192.0	39.68	0.19
	1.00	c							
cooked, no salt	100.0	g	32	3.0	6.3	23.00	278.0	57.00	0.31
	62.00	g	20	1.9	3.9	14.26	172.3	35.34	0.19
	0.50	c							

lettuce

green,raw	100.0	g	31	3.0	6.1	23.00	300.0	62.00	0.30
	64.00	g	20	1.9	3.9	14.72	192.0	39.68	0.19
	1.00	c							
cooked, no salt	100.0	g	32	3.0	6.3	23.00	278.0	57.00	0.31
	62.00	g	20	1.9	3.9	14.26	172.4	35.34	0.19
	0.50	c							
green,raw	100.0	g	31	3.0	6.1	23.00	300.0	62.00	0.30
	64.00	g	20	1.9	3.9	14.72	192.0	39.68	0.19
	1.00	c							
cooked, no salt	100.0	g	32	3.0	6.3	23.00	278.0	57.00	0.31
	62.00	g	20	1.9	3.9	14.26	172.4	35.34	0.19
	0.50	c							
green,raw	100.0	g	31	3.0	6.1	23.00	300.0	62.00	0.30
	64.00	g	20	1.9	3.9	14.72	192.0	39.68	0.19
	1.00	c							
cooked, no salt	100.0	g	32	3.0	6.3	23.00	278.0	57.00	0.31
	62.00	g	20	1.9	3.9	14.26	172.4	35.34	0.19
	0.50	c							

Brussel Sprouts

raw	100.0	g	43	33	9.0	25.00	389.0	69.00	0.30
	88.00	g	38	3.0	7.9	22.00	342.0	60.70	0.26
	1.00	c							

Cabbage

Cabbage	SERVING QUANTITY	SERVING UNIT	CALORIES (kCal)	PROTEIN (g)	TOTAL CARBOHYDRATES (g)	SODIUM (mg)	POTASSIUM (mg)	PHOSPHORUS (mg)	TOTAL FAT (g)
green, chopped	100.0	g	25	1.3	5.8	18.00	170.0	26.00	
	89.00	g	22	1.1	5.2	16.02	151.3	23.14	
	1.00	c							
green shredded, sliced	100.0	g	25	1.3	5.8	18.00	170.0	26.00	
	87.50	g	22	1.1	5.1	15.75	148.7	22.75	
	1.25	c							
green, shredded, boiled, drained, no salt added	100.0	g	23	1.3	5.5	8.00	196.0	33.00	
	75.00	g	17	1.0	4.1	6.00	147.0	24.75	
	0.50	c							
chinese, shredded, raw	100.0	g							
	76.00	g	12	0.9		6.84	181.0	22.04	
	1.00	c							
chinese, cooked, no salt	100.0	g							
	75.00	g	17	1.0		6.00	147.0	24.75	
	0.50	c							
red, shredded	100.00	g	31	1.4	7.4	27.00	243.0	30.00	
	87.50	g	27	1.3	6.5	23.63	212.6	26.25	
	1.25	c							
red, shredded, boiled, drained, no salt added	100.0	g	29	1.5	6.9	28.00	262.0	33.00	
	75.00	g	27	1.1	5.2	21.00	196.5	24.75	
	0.50	c							
Bok Choy or White Mustard, shredded	100.0	g	13	1.5	2.2	65.00	252.0	37.00	
	87.50	g	11	1.3	1.9	56.88	220.5	32.38	
	1.25	c							
Bok Choy/ Pak Choi, shredded, boiled, drained	100.0	g	12	1.6	1.8	34.00	371.0	29.00	
	85.00	g	10	1.3	1.5	28.90	315.3	24.65	
	0.50	c							
Kimchi	100.0	g	15	1.1	2.4	498.00	151.0	24.00	
	150.0	g	23	1.7	3.6	747.00	226.5	36.00	
	1.00	c							

Asparagus	SERVING QUANTITY	SERVING UNIT	CALORIES (kCal)	PROTEIN (g)	TOTAL CARBOHYDRATES (g)	SODIUM (mg)	POTASSIUM (mg)	PHOSPHORUS (mg)	TOTAL FAT (g)
boiled, drained	100.0	g	22	2.4	4.1	14.00	224.0	54.00	0.22
	90.00	g	20	2.2	3.7	12.60	201.6	48.60	0.20
	0.50	c							
frozen	100.0	g	24	3.2	4.1	8.00	253.0	64.00	0.23
	87.00	g	21	2.8	3.6	6.96	220.1	55.68	0.20
	6.00	pcs							
frozen, boiled, drained	100.0	g	18	3.0	1.9	3.00	172.0	49.00	0.42
	90.00	g	16	2.7	1.7	2.70	154.8	44.10	0.38
	0.50	c							
canned, drained	100.0	g	19	2.1	2.5	287.00	172.0	43.00	0.65
	121.0	g	23	2.6	3.0	347.27	208.1	52.03	0.79
	0.50	c							

Cucumber	SERVING QUANTITY	SERVING UNIT	CALORIES (kCal)	PROTEIN (g)	TOTAL CARBOHYDRATES (g)	SODIUM (mg)	POTASSIUM (mg)	PHOSPHORUS (mg)	TOTAL FAT (g)
sliced, raw	100.0	g	15	0.7	3.6	2.00	147.0	24.00	0.11
	52.00	g	8	0.3	1.9	1.04	76.44	12.48	0.06
	0.50	c							
sliced	100.	g	15	0.7	3.6	2.00	147.0	24.00	0.11
sliced, raw	78.00	g	12	0.5	2.8	1.56	114.7	18.72	0.09
	100.0	g			15	0.7	3.6	2.00	147.00

Okra	SERVING QUANTITY	SERVING UNIT	CALORIES (kCal)	PROTEIN (g)	TOTAL CARBOHYDRATES (g)	SODIUM (mg)	POTASSIUM (mg)	PHOSPHORUS (mg)	TOTAL FAT (g)
raw	100.0	g	33	1.9	7.5	7.00	299.0	61.00	0.19
	75.00	g	25	1.5	5.6	5.25	224.3	45.75	0.14
	0.75	c							
sliced, boiled, drained, n.s.	100.0	g	22	1.9	4.5	6.00	135.0	32.00	0.21
	80.00	g	18	1.5	3.6	4.80	108.0	25.60	0.17
	0.50	c							
frozen	100.0	g	30	1.7	6.6	3.00	211.0	42.00	0.25
	85.05	g	26	1.4	5.6	2.55	179.4	35.72	0.21
	3.00	oz							
frozen, boiled, drained, no salt sliced	100.0	g	29	1.6	6.4	3.00	184.0	37.00	0.24
	92.00	g	27	1.5	5.9	2.76	169.3	34.04	0.22
	0.50	c							

Foods to Limit

- Starchy Vegetables (Potatoes, Corn)
  - Nutrition (per 1 medium potato):
    - Calories: 163
    - Protein: 4g
    - Carbohydrates: 37g
    - Fat: 0g
  - Reason: Higher in carbohydrates, which can spike blood sugar levels.
- Canned Vegetables with Added Sugars or Sodium
  - Nutrition (per 1 cup canned corn):
    - Calories: 132
    - Protein: 5g
    - Carbohydrates: 30g
    - Fat: 2g
  - Reason: Often contain added sugars and preservatives that can be detrimental to health.

Proteins

•

Egg

Egg	SERVING QUANTITY	SERVING UNIT	CALORIES (kCal)	PROTEIN (g)	TOTAL CARBOHYDRATES (g)	SODIUM (mg)	POTASSIUM (mg)	PHOSPHORUS (mg)	TOTAL FAT (g)
chicken, raw, large	100.0	g	143	12	0.7	142.00	138.0	198.0	9.51
	50.00	g	72	6.3	0.4	71.00	69.00	99.00	4.76
	1.00	pc							
chicken, fried, large	100.0	g	196	13	0.8	207.00	152.0	215.0	14.84
	46.00	g	90	6.3	0.4	95.22	69.92	98.90	6.83
	1.00	pc							
chicken, poached, large	100.0	g	143	12.5	0.7	297.00	138.0	197.0	9.47
	50.00	g	72	6.3	0.4	148.50	69.00	98.50	4.74
	1.00	pc							
chicken, hard boiled, large	100.0	g	155	12	1.1	124.00	126.0	172.0	10.61
	50.00	g	78	6.3	0.6	62.00	63.00	86.00	5.31
	1.00	pc							
scrambled, fast food	100.0	g	212	14	2.1	187.00	147.0	242.0	16.18
	94.00	g	199	13	2.0	175.78	138.2	227.5	15.21
	2.00	pc							
substitute, liquid	100.0	g	84	12	0.6	177.00	330.0	121.0	3.31
	251.0	g	211	30	1.6	444.27	828.3	303.7	8.31
	1.00	c							
substitute, powder	100.0	g	443	56	21.8	798.19	742.3	476.9	12.97
	9.92	g	44	5.5	2.2	79.20	73.66	47.32	1.29
	0.35	oz							
substitute, frozen	100.0	g	160	11.3	3.2	199.00	213.0	72.00	11.11
	60.00	g	96	6.8	1.9	119.40	127.8	43.20	6.67
	0.25	c							
chicken, egg whites only, raw large egg	100.0	g	52	11	0.7	166.00	163.0	15.00	0.17
	33.00	g	17	3.6	0.2	54.78	53.79	4.95	0.06
	1.00	pc							
chicken, yolk only, raw large egg	100.0	g	322	15.9	3.6	48.00	109.0	390.0	26.54
	17.00	g	55	2.7	0.6	8.16	18.53	66.30	4.51
	1.00	pc							
chicken, whole, raw, frozen	100.0	g	147	12	1.0	128.00	135.0	193.0	9.95
	56.70	g	83	7.0	0.6	72.57	76.54	109.4	5.64
	2.00	oz							
yolk only, frozen, raw	100.0	g	296	15.5	0.8	67.00	121.0	419.9	25.60
	56.70	g	168	8.8	0.5	37.99	68.61	238.1	14.51
	2.00	oz							
whites, frozen, raw	100.0	g	48	10	1.0	169.00	169.0	13.00	0.00
	56.70	g	27	5.8	0.6	95.82	95.82	7.37	0.00
	2.00	oz							
duck, raw	100.0	g	185	13	1.5	146.00	222.0	220.0	13.77
	70.00	g	130	9.0	1.0	102.20	155.4	154.0	9.64
	1.00	pc							
quail, raw	100.0	g	158	13.1	0.4	141.00	132.0	226.0	11.09
	9.00	g	14	1.2	0.0	12.69	11.88	20.34	1.00
	1.00	pc							

Chicken	SERVING QUANTITY	SERVING UNIT	CALORIES (KCal)	PROTEIN (g)	TOTAL CARBOHYDRATES (g)	SODIUM (mg)	POTASSIUM (mg)	PHOSPHORUS (mg)	TOTAL FAT (g)
ground, raw	100.0	g	143	17.4	0.0	60.00	522.0	178.0	8.10
meat and skin, raw	100.0	g	215	18	0.0	70.00	189.0	147.0	15.06
	113.0	g	244	21.1	0.0	79.38	214.3	166.7	17.08
	4.00	oz							
meat and skin, roasted	100.0	g	239	27	0.0	82.00	223.0	182.0	13.60
	85.05	g	203	23	0.0	69.74	189.7	154.8	11.57
	3.00	oz							
thigh meat only, fried	100.0	g	218	28	1.2	95.00	259.0	199.0	10.30
	85.05	g	185	24	1.0	80.80	220.3	169.3	8.76
	3.00	oz							
thigh meat only, roasted	100.0	g	179	24	0.0	106.00	269.0	230.0	8.15
	85.05	g	152	21.1	0.0	90.15	228.8	195.61	6.93
	3.00	oz							
wing meat only, fried	100.0	g	211	30	0.0	91.00	208.0	164.0	9.15
	85.05	g	179	25	0.0	77.39	176.9	139.5	7.78
	3.00	oz							
wing meat only, roasted	100.0	g	203	30	0.0	92.00	210.0	166.0	8.13
	85.05	g	173	26	0.0	78.25	178.6	141.18	6.91
	3.00	oz							
wing meat only, stewed	100.0	g	181	27	0.0	73.00	153.0	134.0	7.18
	85.05	g	154	23	0.0	62.09	130.1	113.97	6.11
	3.00	oz							
back meat only, fried	100.0	g	288	30	5.7	99.00	251.0	176.0	4.12
	85.05	g	245	25	4.8	84.20	213.5	149.7	3.50
	3.00	oz							
back meat only, roasted	100.0	g	239	28	0.0	96.00	237.0	165.0	13.16
	85.05	g	203	24	0.0	81.65	201.5	140.3	11.19
	3.00	oz							
back meat only, stewed	100.0	g	209	25	0.0	67.00	158.0	130.0	11.19
	85.05	g	178	21.5	0.0	56.98	134.3 8	110.5 6	9.52
	3.00	oz							
drumstick meat only, fried	100.0	g	195	28	0.0	96.00	249.0	186.0	8.08
	85.05	g	166	24	0.0	81.65	211.77	158.2	6.87
	3.00	oz							
drumstick meat only, roasted	100.0	g	155	24	0.0	128.00	256.0	200.0	5.70
	85.05	g	132	20	0.0	108.86	217.7	170.1	4.85
	3	oz							

Chicken	SERVING QUANTITY	SERVING UNIT	CALORIES (kCal)	PROTEIN (g)	TOTAL CARBOHYDRATES (g)	SODIUM (mg)	POTASSIUM (mg)	PHOSPHORUS (mg)	TOTAL FAT (g)
drumstick meat only, stewed	100.0	g	169	27	0.0	80.00	199.0	150.0	5.71
	85.05	g	144	23	0.0	68.04	169.2	127.57	4.86
	3.00	oz							
leg meat only, fried	100.0	g	208	28	0.7	96.00	254.0	193.0	9.32
	85.05	g	177	24	0.6	81.65	216.0	164.1	7.93
	3.00	oz							
leg meat only, roasted	100.0	g	174	24	0.0	99.00	269.0	205.0	7.80
	85.05	g	148	20	0.0	84.20	228.8	174.4	6.63
	3.00	oz							
leg meat only, stewed	100.0	g	185	26	0.0	78.00	190.0	149.0	8.06
	85.05	g	157	22	0.0	66.34	161.59	126.7	6.85
	3.00	oz							
pate, chicken liver, canned	100.0	g	201	13.5	6.6	386.00	95.00	175.0	13.10
	52.00	g	105	7.0	3.4	200.72	49.40	91.00	6.81
	4.00	tbsp							
chicken tenders, fast food	100.0	g	271	19	17.3	769.00	373.0	282.0	13.95
	62.00	g	168	11.9	10.7	476.78	231.2	174.8	8.65
	4.00	pcs							
chicken patty, frozen, cooked	100.0	g	287	14.9	12.8	532.00	261.0	208.0	19.58
bratwurst, chicken, cooked	100.0	g	176	19	0.0	72.00	211.0	160.0	10.30
	83.92	g	148	16.	0.0	60.42	177.1	134.3	8.69
	2.96	oz							
sausage, chicken/beef, smoked	100.0	g	295	18.5	0.0	1,020	139.0	111.00	244.00
	138.0	g	251	15.7	0.0	867.51	118.2	94.41	20.41
	1.00	c							

Turkey

Turkey	SERVING QUANTITY	SERVING UNIT	CALORIES (kCal)	PROTEIN (g)	TOTAL CARBOHYDRATES (g)	SODIUM (mg)	POTASSIUM (mg)	PHOSPHORUS (mg)	TOTAL FAT (g)
breast, meat & skin, raw	100.0	g	144	21	0.1	112.00	224.0	183.0	5.64
	113.4	g	163	24	0.2	127.01	254.0	207.5	6.40
	4.00	oz							
breast, meat & skin, roasted	100.0	g	189	28	0.1	103.00	239.0	223.0	7.39
	85.05	g	161	24	0.1	87.60	203.3	189.7	6.29
	3.00	oz							
breast, meat only, raw	100.0	g	114	23	0.0	74.00	267.0	185.0	2.33
	85.05	g	97	20	0.0	62.94	227.1	157.3	1.98
	3.00	oz							
breast, meat only, roasted	100.0	g	136	29	0.0	114.00	297.0	253.0	1.97
	85.05	g	116	25.1	0.0	96.96	252.6	215.17	1.68
	3.00	oz							
ground, raw	100.0	g	148	20	0.0	58.00	237.0	200.0	7.66
	113.4	g	168	22	0.0	65.77	268.7	226.8	8.69
	4.00	oz							
ground, cooked	100.0	g	203	27	0.0	78.00	294.0	254.0	10.40
	85.05	g	173	23	0.0	66.34	250.0	216.0	8.85
	3.00	oz							
white rotisserie, deli cut	100.0	g	112	13.5	7.7	1,200	349.0	158.0	3.00
	56.70	g	64	7.7	4.4	680.40	197.9	89.59	1.70
	2.00	oz							
ham, extra lean, sliced	100.0	g	134	19	0.9	1,038	299.0	304.0	5.80
	20.00	g	27	3.9	0.2	207.60	59.80	60.80	1.16
	1.00	pc							
pastrami, sliced	100.0	g	139	16	3.3	1,123.0	345.0	200.0	6.21
	56.70	g	79	9.2	1.9	636.74	195.6	113.4	3.52
	2.00	slices							
bologna	100.0	g	209	11.4	4.7	1,071.0	135.0	114.0	16.05
	56.70	g	119	6.5	2.7	607.26	76.55	64.64	9.10
	2.00	slices							
salami	100.0	g	172	19	1.6	1,107.0	216.0	266.0	9.21
	56.70	g	98	11	0.9	627.67	122.5	150.8	5.22
	2.00	slices							
bacon, turkey, cooked	100.0	g	382	29	3.1	2,285	395.0	460.0	27.90
	28.35	g	108	8.4	0.9	647.80	111.98	130.4	7.91
	1.00	oz							
bacon, turkey, low sodium	100.0	g	253	13	4.8	900.00	156.0	145.0	20.0
	15.00	g	38	2.0	0.7	135.00	23.40	21.75	3.00
	1.00	svg							
sausage, turkey, cooked	100.0	g	196	24	0.0	665.00	298.0	202.0	10.4
	56.70	g	111	13	0.0	377.06	168.9	114.53	5.92
	2.00	oz							

Salmon	SERVING QUANTITY	SERVING UNIT	CALORIES (kCal)	PROTEIN (g)	TOTAL CARBOHYDRATES (g)	SODIUM (mg)	POTASSIUM (mg)	PHOSPHORUS (mg)	TOTAL FAT (g)
pink, raw	100.0	g	127	20	0.0	74.99	365.9	260.9	4.40
	113.4	g	144	2	0.0	85.04	415.0	295.9	4.99
	4.00	oz							
atlantic, wild, raw	100.0	g	142	19	0.0	44.00	489.9	199.9	0.98
	113.4	g	161	22	0.0	49.89	555.6	226.7	1.11
	4.00	oz							
atlantic, farmed,raw	100.0	g	208	20	0.0	58.99	362.9	239.9	13.42
	113.39	g	236	23	0.0	66.90	411.6	272.1	15.22
	4.00	oz							
pink, canned, drained solids, w/ bone	100.0	g	138	23	0.0	380.78	332.8	378.7	5.02
	85.05	g	117	19	0.0	323.85	283.1	322.2	4.27
	3.00	oz							
pink, canned, with bone and liquid no salt	100.0	g	139	19	0.0	75.00	325.9	328.9	6.05
	56.70	g	79	11.2	0.0	42.52	184.8	186.5	3.43
	2.00	oz							
pink, canned, drained solids without skin and bones	100.0	g	136	24	0.0	378.00	326.0	253.0	4.21
	85.05	g	116	21	0.0	321.49	277.3	215.2	3.58
	3.00	oz							
chum, canned, drained, with bone no salt	100.0	g	141	21.4	0.0	75.00	300.0	353.9	5.50
	56.70	g	80	12	0.0	42.52	170.1	200.7	3.12
	2.00	oz							
nuggets, breaded, frozen, heated	100.0	g	212	12.7	14.0	173.00	165.0	176.0	11.72
Sardines									
spanish	100.0	g	212	6.2	14.2	310.00	0.00	na	14.16
	113.00	g	240	7.0	16.0	350.00	0.00	na	16.00
	4.00	oz							
atlantic, canned in oil, with bones	100.0	g	208	24	0.0	307.00	397.0	490.0	11.45
	24.00	g	50	5.9	0.0	73.68	95.28	117.6	2.75
	2.00	oz							
portuguese	100.0	g	236	25	0.0	500.00	na	na	12.73
	55.00	g	130	14.0	0.0	275.00	na	na	7.00
	0.50	c							
fillets, canned	100.0	g	338	18	7.3	364.00	na	na	26.36
	55.00	g	186	10	4.0	200.00	na	na	14.50
	0.25	c							

Herring	SERVING QUANTITY	SERVING UNIT	CALORIES (kCal)	PROTEIN (g)	TOTAL CARBOHYDRATES (g)	SODIUM (mg)	POTASSIUM (mg)	PHOSPHORUS (mg)	TOTAL FAT (g)
Pacific, raw	100.0	g	195	16.	0.0	73.99	422.9	227.9	13.88
	113.4	g	221	18	0.0	83.91	479.6	258.5	15.74
	4.00	oz							
Atlantic, raw	100.0	g	158	18	0.0	89.99	326.9	235.9	9.04
	113.4	g	179	20	0.0	102.05	370.8	267.6	10.25
	4.00	oz							
Pacific, cooked, dry heat	100.0	g	250	21	0.0	95.00	541.9	292.0	17.79
	85.05	g	213	17.9	0.0	80.80	460.9	248.3	15.13
	3.00	oz							
Atlantic, cooked, dry heat	100.0	g	203	23.	0.0	115.00	419.0	303.0	11.49
	85.05	g	173	19	0.0	97.81	356.3	257.7	9.86
	3.00	oz							
Roe or eggs, Pacific (Alaska Native)	100.0	g	74	9.6	4.5	61.00	na	na	1.93
	85.05	g	63	8.2	3.8	51.88	na	na	1.64
	3.00	oz							

Mackerel

Atlantic or Boston, raw fillet	100.0	g	205	18	0.0	89.99	313.9	216.9	13.89
	113.4	g	232	21.1	0.0	102.05	356.0	246.0	15.75
	4.00	oz							
pacific and Jack, raw fillet	100.0	g	158	20	0.0	85.99	405.9	124.9	7.89
	113.4	g	179	22.	0.0	97.51	460.3	141.71	8.95
	4.00	oz							
Atlantic Spanish, raw fillet	100.0	g	139	19	0.0	58.99	445.9	204.9	6.30
	113.4	g	158	22	0.0	66.90	505.7	232.5	7.14
	4.00	oz							
Jack, canned, solids, drained	100.0	g	156	23	0.0	378.99	194.0	301.0	6.30
	56.70	g	88	13	0.0	214.89	110.0	170.6	3.57
	2.00	oz							
Atlantic or Boston, cooked, dry heat	100.0	g	262	24	0.0	83.00	401.0	278.0	17.81
	85.05	g	223	20	0.0	70.59	341.0	236.4	15.15
	3.00	oz							
Atlantic, Spanish, cooked, dry heat	100.0	g	158	23	0.0	66.00	553.9	271.0	6.32
	85.05	g	134	20	0.0	56.13	471.17	230.5	5.38
	3.00	oz							
Pacific and Jack, mixed species, cooked	100.0	g	201	25	0.0	110.00	520.9	160.0	10.12
	85.05	g	171	22	0.0	93.55	443.1	136.1	8.61
	3.00	oz							

Beans	SERVING QUANTITY	SERVING UNIT	CALORIES (kCal)	PROTEIN (g)	TOTAL CARBOHYDRATES (g)	SODIUM (mg)	POTASSIUM (mg)	PHOSPHORUS (mg)	TOTAL FAT (g)
Lentils/Pinto /Navy	100.0	g	131	8.6	23.9	1.67	398.9	165.7	0.49
	92.00	g	121	8.0	22.0	1.54	367.0	152.5	0.45
	0.50	c							
Lima	100.0	g	113	6.8	20.2	8.00	467.0	136.0	0.86
	78.00	g	88	5.3	15.7	6.24	364.2	106.1	0.67
	0.50	c							
Broad or Fava	100.0	g	72	5.6	11.7	50.00	250.0	95.00	0.60
	81.75	g	59	4.6	9.6	40.88	204.4	77.66	0.49
	0.75	c							
Black beans, boiled	100.0	g	132	8.9	23.7	1.00	355.0	140.0	0.54
	86.00	g	114	7.6	20.4	0.86	305.3	120.4	0.46
	0.50	c							
Mungo, boiled	100.0	g	105	7.5	18.3	7.00	231.0	156.0	0.55
	90.00	g	95	6.8	16.5	6.30	207.9	140.4	0.50
	0.50	c							
sprouts, Mung	100.0	g	30	3.0	5.9	6.00	149.0	54.00	0.18
	78.00	g	23	2.4	4.6	4.68	116.2	42.12	0.14
	0.75	c							
Kidney, boiled	100.0	g	127	8.7	22.8	1.00	405.0	138.0	0.50
	88.50	g	112	7.7	20.2	0.89	358.4	122.13	0.44
	0.50	c							
Navy, boiled	100.0	g	140	8.2	26.1	0.00	389.0	144.0	0.62
	91.00	g	127	7.5	23.7	0.00	353.9	131.0	0.56
	0.50	c							
Lupin, boiled	100.0	g	119	15.6	9.9	4.00	245.0	128.0	2.92
	83.00	g	99	12.	8.2	3.32	203.3	106.2	2.42
	0.50	c							
Pinto, frozen	100.0	g	170	9.8	32.5	92.00	755.9	117.0	0.50
	94.49	g	161	9.3	31.0	86.93	714.3	110.55	0.47
	3.33	oz							
Pinto, boiled	100.0	g	143	9.0	26.2	1.00	436.0	147.0	0.65
	85.50	g	122	7.7	22.4	0.86	372.8	125.7	0.56
	0.50	c							
White (Cannellini), boiled no salt	100.0	g	139	9.7	25.1	6.00	561.0	113.0	0.35
	89.50	g	124	8.7	22.5	5.37	502.1	101.14	0.31
	0.50	c							

Beans	Serving Quantity	Serving Unit	Calories (kcal)	Protein (g)	Total Carbohydrates (g)	Sodium (mg)	Potassium (mg)	Phosphorus (mg)	Total Fat (g)
White, small, boiled, no salt	100.0	g	142	9.0	25.8	2.00	463.0	169.0	0.64
	89.50	g	127	8.0	23.1	1.79	414.4	151.26	0.57
	0.50	c							
sprouts, Kidney	100.0	g	29	4.2	4.1	6.00	187.0	37.00	0.50
	92.00	g	27	3.9	3.8	5.52	172.0	34.04	0.46
	0.50	c							
sprouts, Navy	100.0	g	67	6.2	13.1	13.00	307.0	100.0	0.70
	78.00	g	52	4.8	10.2	10.14	239.5	78.00	0.55
	0.75	c							
sprouts, Pinto	100.0	g	62	5.3	11.6	153.00	307.0	94.00	0.90
	85.05	g	53	4.5	9.9	130.12	262.1	79.95	0.77
	3.00	oz							
French, boiled	100.0	g	129	7.1	24.0	6.00	370.0	102.0	0.76
	88.50	g	114	6.2	21.3	5.31	327.4	90.27	0.67
	0.50	c							
baked, prepared	100.0	g	155	5.5	21.6	422.00	358.0	109.0	5.15
	126.5	g	196	7.0	27.4	533.83	452.8	138.0	6.51
	0.50	c							
Refried, canned	100.0	g	90	5.0	13.6	370.00	319.0	92.00	2.01
	119.0	g	107	5.9	16.1	440.30	379.6	109.5	2.39
	0.50	c							

Chickpeas

Chickpeas	Serving Quantity	Serving Unit	Calories (kcal)	Protein (g)	Total Carbohydrates (g)	Sodium (mg)	Potassium (mg)	Phosphorus (mg)	Total Fat (g)
garbanzos/ bengal gram, canned	100.0	g	88	4.9	13.5	278.00	144.0	80.00	1.95
	120.0	g	106	5.9	16.2	333.60	172.8	96.00	2.34
	0.50	c							
garbanzos/ bengal gram, boiled	100.0	g	164	8.9	27.4	7.00	291.0	168.0	2.59
	82.00	g	134	7.3	22.5	5.74	238.6	137.8	2.12
	0.50	c							
garbanzos/ bengal gram, canned drained, rinsed in tap water	100.0	g	138	7.0	22.9	212.00	109.0	80.00	2.47
	152.0	g	210	10	34.8	322.24	165.7	121.6	3.75
	1.00	c							
garbanzos/ bengal gram, canned low sodium	100	g	88	4.9	13.5	132.00	144.0	80.00	1.95
	240	g	211	11.8	32.4	316.80	345.6	192.0	4.68
	1	c							
flour	100.0	g	387	22	57.8	64.00	846.0	318.0	6.69
	92.00	g	110	6.4	16.4	18.14	239.8	90.15	1.90
	1.00	c							

Tofu

	SERVING QUANTITY	SERVING UNIT	CALORIES (kCal)	PROTEIN (g)	TOTAL CARBOHYDRATES (g)	SODIUM (mg)	POTASSIUM (mg)	PHOSPHORUS (mg)	TOTAL FAT (g)
soft with calcium sulfate and magnesium chloride (Nigari)	100.0	g	61	7.2	1.2	8.00	120.0	92.00	3.69
	85.05	g	52	6.1	1.0	6.80	102.1	78.25	3.14
	3.00	oz							
firm with calcium sulfate and magnesium chloride (Nigari)	100.0	g	78	9.0	2.9	12.00	148.0	121.0	4.17
	85.05	g	66	7.7	2.4	10.21	125.9	102.9	3.55
	3.00	oz							
silken tofu (Vitasoy USA)	100.0	g	43	4.8	0.6	2.00	na	na	2.40
	91.00	g	39	4.4	0.5	1.82	na	na	2.18
	0.20	package							

Tempeh

raw	100.0	g	192	20	7.6	9.00	412.0	266.0	10.80
	83.00	g	159	16	6.3	7.47	341.9	220.8	8.96
	0.50	c							
cooked	100.0	g	185	20	7.6	14.00	401.0	253.0	11.38

Edamame

frozen, unprepared	100.0	g	109	11.2	7.6	6.00	482.0	161.0	4.73
	118.0	g	129	13	9.0	7.08	568.7	189.9	5.58
	1.00	c							
frozen, prepared	100.0	g	121	11.9	8.9	6.00	436.0	261.9	5.20
	155.00	g	188	18.5	13.8	9.30	675.80	169.00	8.06
	1	c							

Spirulina

seaweed, fresh/ raw	100.0	g	26	5.9	2.4	98.00	127.0	11.00	0.39
	28.35	g	7	1.7	0.7	27.78	36.00	3.12	0.11
	1.00	oz							
seaweed, dried	100.0	g	290	57	23.9	1,048	1363	118.0	7.72
	112.0	g	325	64	26.8	1,173.8	1526	132.1	8.65
	1.00	c							

Foods to Limit

- Processed Meats (Sausages, Hot Dogs)
    - Nutrition (per 1 link sausage):
        - Calories: 300
        - Protein: 12g
        - Carbohydrates: 2g
        - Fat: 28g
    - Reason: Often high in unhealthy fats, sodium, and preservatives.
- High-Fat Dairy Products (Cream, Full-Fat Cheese)
    - Nutrition (per 1 oz cheddar cheese):
        - Calories: 113
        - Protein: 7g
        - Carbohydrates: 1g
        - Fat: 9g
    - Reason: Can contribute to inflammation and weight gain.

Grains

Grains are a source of energy for the cells, therefore are not completely contraindicated in your diet. However, our individual tolerance to carbs vary from one person to another. Thus, we need to take grains with caution and in moderation, to control any blood sugar spikes so as not to aggravate any ongoing insulin resistance. Find the grain that your body can tolerate well.

Quinoa	SERVING QUANTITY	SERVING UNIT	CALORIES (kCal)	PROTEIN (g)	TOTAL CARBOHYDRATES (g)	SODIUM (mg)	POTASSIUM (mg)	PHOSPHORUS (mg)	TOTAL FAT (g)
cooked	100.0	g	120	4.4	21.3	7.00	172.0	152.0	1.92
	185.0	g	222	8.1	39.4	13.00	318.0	281.0	3.55
	1.00	c							
uncooked	100.0	g	368	14.1	64.2	5.00	563.0	457.0	6.07
	170.0	g	626	24.	109.	8.50	957.0	777.0	10.30
	1.00	c							
pasta from quinoa flour (gluten-free) not packed	100.0	g	152	3.2	31.1	4.00	63.00	91.00	2.07
	132.0	g	201	4.3	41.1	5.28	83.20	120.0	2.73
	1.00	c							
Amaranth									
Grain cooked	100.0	g	102	3.8	18.7	6.00	135.0	148.0	1.58
	246.0	g	251	9.4	46.0	14.80	332.0	364.0	3.89
	1.00	c							
Rice (brown)									
brown, cooked, no salt, no fat	100.0	g	122	2.7	25.5				
	196.0	g	239	5.4	49.9	5.00	75.00	94.00	1.30
	1.00	c							
wild, cooked	100.0	g	101	4.0	21.3	5.00	20.00	33.00	0.27
	164.0	g	166	6.5	35.0	6.60	26.40	43.60	0.36
	1.00	c							

CAUTION: Still high in Carbs, consume moderately

Foods to Limit

- Refined Grains (White Bread, White Rice)
    - Nutrition (per 1 slice white bread):
        - Calories: 66
        - Protein: 2g
        - Carbohydrates: 13g
        - Fat: 1g
    - Reason: Low in nutrients and fiber, leading to rapid blood sugar spikes.
- Sugary Cereals
    - Nutrition (per 1 cup sugary cereal):
        - Calories: 150
        - Protein: 2g
        - Carbohydrates: 30g
        - Fat: 2g
    - Reason: High in added sugars and low in fiber, contributing to insulin resistance.

Fails

Avocado	SERVING QUANTITY	SERVING UNIT	CALORIES (kCal)	PROTEIN (g)	TOTAL CARBOHYDRATES (g)	SODIUM (mg)	POTASSIUM (mg)	PHOSPHORUS (mg)	TOTAL FAT (g)
fresh, raw mashed/ pureed	100.0	g	160	2.0	8.5	7.00	485.0	52.00	14.66
	230.0	g	368	4.6	19.6	16.10	1,120	120.0	33.70
	1.00	c							
oil	100.0	g	884	0.0	0.0	0.00	0.00	0.00	100.00
	14.00	g	124	0.0	0.0	0.00	0.00	0.00	14.00
	1.00	tbsp							
dressing	100.0	g	427	1.9	7.4	867.00	58.00	31.00	43.33
	15.30	g	65	0.3	1.1	133.00	8.87	4.74	6.63
	1.00	tbsp							
California, raw/fresh no seed and skin	100.0	g	167	2.0	8.6	8.00	507.0	54.00	15.41
	136.0	g	227	2.7	11.8	10.90	690.0	73.40	21.00
	1.00	pc/ item							
Florida, fresh/ raw no seed and skin	100.0	g	120	2.2	7.8	2.00	351.0	40.00	10.06
	304.0	g	365	6.8	23.8	6.08	1,070	122.0	30.60
	1.00	pc/ item							
Guacamole	100.0	g	155	2.0	8.5	344.00	472.0	51.00	14.18
	15.00	G	23	0.3	1.3	51.60	70.80	7.65	2.13
	1.00	tbsp							
Olive									
oil, extra virgin, virgin	100	g	884	0.0	0.0	2.00	1.00	0.00	100.0
	14	g	124	0.0	0.0	0.28	0.14	0.00	14.0
	1	tbsp							
black, kalamata	100	g	116	0.8	6.0	735.00	8.00	3.00	10.9
	15	g	17	0.1	0.9	110.00	1.20	0.45	1.6
	3	pcs							
green	100	g	145	1.0	3.8	1556	42.00	4.00	15.3
	15	g	22	0.2	0.6	233.00	6.30	0.60	2.3
	3	pcs							
spread (tapenade)	100	g	278	0.7	4.2	835.00	17.00	3.00	30.1
	16	g	45	0.1	0.7	134.00	2.72	0.48	4.8
	1	tbsp							
stuffed	100	g	128	1.0	4.0	1340	58.00	6.00	13.2
	15	g	19	0.2	0.6	201.00	8.70	0.90	2.0
	3	pcs							
Poppyseed									
oil	100	g	884	0.0	0.0	0.00	0.00	0.00	100.0
	13.6	g	120	0.0	0.0	0.00	0.00	0.00	13.6
	1	tbsp							
salad dressing, creamy	100	g	399	0.9	23.7	933.00	61.00	49.00	33.3
	33	g	132	0.3	7.8	307.89	20.13	16.17	11.0
	2	tbsp							

Almond

	SERVING QUANTITY	SERVING UNIT	CALORIES (kCal)	PROTEIN (g)	TOTAL CARBOHYDRATES (g)	SODIUM (mg)	POTASSIUM (mg)	PHOSPHORUS (mg)	TOTAL FAT (g)
whole	100	g	579	21	21.6	1.00	733.0	481.0	49.9
	35.75	g	207	7.6	7.7	0.36	262.1	171.96	17.9
	0.25	c							
slivered	100	g	579	21	21.6	1.00	733.0	481.0	49.9
	27	g	156	5.7	5.8	0.27	197.91	129.	13.5
	0.25	c							
ground	100	g	579	21	21.6	1.00	733	481.0	49.9
	23.75	g	138	5.0	5.1	0.24	174.1	114.4	11.9
	0.25	c							
paste (marzipan)	100	g	458	9.0	47.8	9.00	314.0	258.0	27.7
	28.38	g	130	2.6	13.6	2.55	89.10	73.21	7.9
	2	tbsp							
oil	100	g	884	0.0	0.0	0.00	0.00	0.00	100.0
	13.6	g	120	0.0	0.0	0.00	0.00	0.00	13.6
	1	tbsp							
butter, without salt added	100	g	614	21	18.8	227.00	748.0	508.0	55.5
	16	g	98	3.4	3.0	1.12	119.7	81.28	8.9
	1	tbsp							
dry roasted, without salt added	100	g	598	3.0	21.0	3.00	713.0	471.0	52.5
	34.5	g	206	7.2	7.3	1.04	245.9	162.5	18.1
	0.25	c							
oil roasted, without salt	100	g	607	21	17.7	1.00	699.0	466.0	55.2
	39.25	g	238	8.3	6.9	0.39	274.4	182.9	21.7
	0.25	c							
milk, unsweetened, shelf stable	100	g	15	0.4	1.3	72.00	67.00	9.00	1.0
	262	g	39	1.1	3.4	188.64	175.5	23.58	2.5
	1	c							
milk, sweetened, vanilla flavor ready-to-drink	100	g	38	0.4	6.6	63.00	50.00	8.00	1.0
	240	g	91	1.0	15.8	151.20	120.0	19.20	2.5
	1	c							
milk, chocolate flavor, unsweetened fortified Vit. D2 and E	100	g	21	0.8	1.3	75.00	96.00	17.00	1.5
	240	g	50	2.0	3.0	180.00	130.4	40.80	3.5
	1	c							

Coconut

oil	100	g	833	0.0	0.0	0.00	0.00	0.00	99.1
	14	g	117	0.0	0.0	0.00	0.00	0.00	13.9
	1	tbsp							

	SERVING QUANTITY	SERVING UNIT	CALORIES (kCal)	PROTEIN (g)	TOTAL CARBOHYDRATES (g)	SODIUM (mg)	POTASSIUM (mg)	PHOSPHORUS (mg)	TOTAL FAT (g)
Safflower									
oil	100	g	884	0.0	0.0	0.00	0.00	0.00	100.0
	14	g	124	0.0	0.0	0.00	0.00	0.00	14.0
	1	tbsp							
Canola									
oil	100	g	884	0.0	0.0	0.00	0.00	0.00	100.0
	14	g	124	0.0	0.0	0.00	0.00	0.00	14.0
	1	tbsp							
Soybean									
oil	100	g	884	0.0	0.0	0.00	0.00	0.00	100.0
	14	g	124	0.0	0.0	0.00	0.00	0.00	14.0
	1	tbsp							
Butter									
stick	100	g	717	0.9	0.1	643.00	24.00	24.00	81.1
	14	g	100	0.1	0.0	90.00	3.36	3.36	11.4
	1	tbsp							
light, stick or tub	100	g	499	3.3	0.0	450.00	71.00	34.00	55.1
	14	g	70	0.5	0.0	63.00	9.94	4.76	7.7
	1	tbsp							
unsalted	100	g	717	0.9	0.1	11.00	24.00	24.00	81.1
	14	g	102	0.1	0.0	1.56	3.41	3.41	11.5
	1	tbsp							
Peanut									
oil	100	g	884	0.0	0.0	0.00	0.00	0.00	100.0
	13.5	g	119	0.0	0.0	0.00	0.00	0.00	13.5
	1	tbsp							
Hazelnut									
oil	100	g	884	0.0	0.0	0.00	0.00	0.00	100.0
	13.6	g	120	0.0	0.0	0.00	0.00	0.00	13.6
	1	tbsp							
whole (1 oz= 21 kernels)	100	g	628	15	16.7	0.00	680.0	290.0	60.8
	33.75	g	212	5.1	5.6	0.00	229.5	97.88	20.5
	0.25	c							
blanched	100	g	629	13.7	17.0	0.00	658.0	310.0	61.2
	28.35	g	178	3.9	4.8	0.00	186.5	87.89	17.3
	1	oz							
chopped	100	g	628	15	16.7	0.00	680.0	290.0	60.8
	28.75	g	181	4.3	4.8	0.00	195.5	83.38	17.5
	0.25	c							

	SERVING QUANTITY	SERVING UNIT	CALORIES (kCal)	PROTEIN (g)	TOTAL CARBOHYDRATES (g)	SODIUM (mg)	POTASSIUM (mg)	PHOSPHORUS (mg)	TOTAL FAT (g)
Acorn									
Nuts	100	g	387	6.2	40.8	0.00	539.0	79.00	23.9
	28.35	g	110	1.7	11.6	0.00	152.8	22.40	6.8
	1	oz							
flour	100	g	501	7.5	54.7	0.00	712.0	103.0	30.2
	28.35	g	142	2.1	15.5	0.00	201.8	29.20	8.6
	1	oz							
nuts, dried	100	g	509	8.1	53.7	0.00	709.0	103.0	31.4
	28.35	g	144	2.3	15.2	0.00	201.0	29.20	8.9
	1	oz							
Chia									
seeds, dried	100	g	486	16.5	42.1	16.00	407.0	860.0	30.7
	28.35	g	138	4.7	11.9	4.54	115.4	243.8	8.7
	1	oz							
Hemp									
seeds, hulled	100	g	553	31	8.7	5.00	1,200	1,650	48.8
	30	g	166	9.5	2.6	1.50	360.0	495.0	14.6
	3	tbsp							
Flaxseed									
seeds, whole	100	g	534	18	28.9	30.00	813.0	642.0	42.2
	10.3	g	55	1.9	3.0	3.09	83.70	66.10	4.3
	1	tbsp							
seeds, ground	7	g	37	1.3	2.0	2.10	56.90	44.90	3.0
	1	tbsp							
oil	100	g	884	0.1	0.0	0.00	0.00	1.00	100.0
	14	g	124	0.0	0.0	0.00	0.00	0.14	14.0
	1	tbsp							
oil with added sliced flaxseed	100	g	878	0.4	0.4	6.00	31.00	27.00	99.0
	13.7	g	120	0.1	0.1	0.82	4.25	3.70	13.6
	1	tbsp							
oil, cold pressed	100	g	884	0.1	0.0	0.00	0.00	1.00	100.0
	13.6	g	120	0.0	0.0	0.00	0.00	0.14	13.6
	1	tbsp							
Pumpkin									
meat, 1" cubes	100	g	26	1.0	6.5	1.00	340.0	44.00	0.1
	116	g	30	1.2	7.5	1.16	394.4	51.04	0.1
	1	c							
flowers	100	g	15	1.0	3.3	5.00	173.0	49.00	0.1
	33	g	1	0.0	0.1	0.20	6.92	1.96	0.0
	1	c							
meat, boiled, drained, no salt added	100	g	20	0.7	4.9	1.00	230.0	30.00	0.1
	122.5	g	25	0.9	6.0	1.23	281.	36.75	0.1
	0.5	c							
pumpkin pie spice powder	100	g	342	5.8	69.3	52.00	663.0	118.0	12.6
	1.7	g	6	0.1	1.2	0.88	11.27	2.01	0.2
	1	tsp							

Foods to Limit

- Trans Fats (Partially Hydrogenated Oils)
    - Nutrition (per 1 tablespoon margarine):
        - Calories: 100
        - Protein: 0g
        - Carbohydrates: 0g
        - Fat: 11g
    - Reason: Linked to inflammation and increased risk of heart disease.
- High-Saturated Fat Foods (Butter, Lard)
    - Nutrition (per 1 tablespoon butter):
        - Calories: 102
        - Protein: 0g
        - Carbohydrates: 0g
        - Fat: 12g
    - Reason: Can contribute to weight gain and hormonal imbalances.

By focusing on whole, nutrient-dense foods and limiting processed options, you can create a balanced diet that supports your health and fertility. This ultimate PCOS food list serves as a guide to help you make informed choices that align with your wellness goals.

Chapter 5: Sample Recipes for Every Meal

Incorporating the right foods into your diet can be both delicious and satisfying. Here are some easy-to-follow recipes for breakfast, lunch, dinner, and snacks that utilize the foods from the PCOS food list, along with their serving sizes and macronutrient information.

BERRY SMOOTHIE BOWL

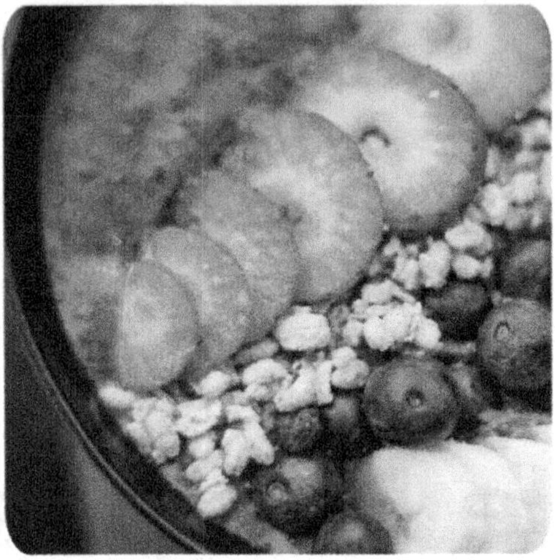

1 bowl

MACROS

- Calories: 300
- Protein: 5g
- Carbohydrates: 50g
- Fat: 10g

INGREDIENTS

- 1 cup mixed berries (blueberries, strawberries, raspberries)
- 1 banana
- 1/2 cup unsweetened almond milk (or any milk of choice)
- 1 tablespoon chia seeds
- Toppings: sliced banana, granola, and a sprinkle of nuts

DIRECTIONS

1. In a blender, combine the mixed berries, banana, almond milk, and chia seeds. Blend until smooth.
2. Pour the smoothie into a bowl and top with sliced banana, granola, and nuts.
3. Enjoy immediately!

SPINACH AND FETA OMELET

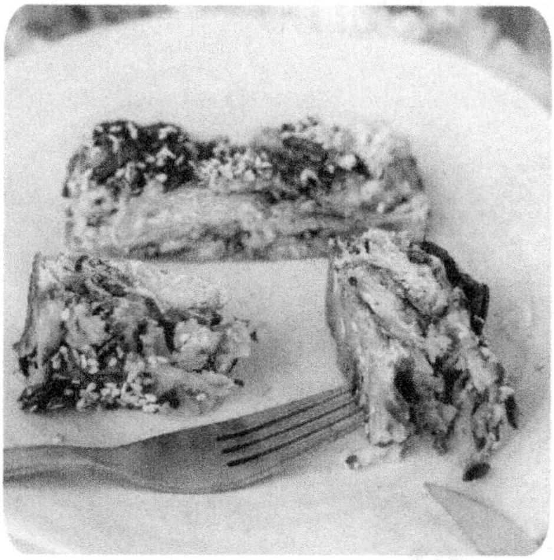

1 omelet

MACROS

- Calories: 200
- Protein: 14g
- Carbohydrates: 2g
- Fat: 15g

INGREDIENTS

- 2 eggs
- 1 cup fresh spinach
- 1/4 cup feta cheese, crumbled
- Salt and pepper to taste
- 1 teaspoon olive oil

DIRECTIONS

1. In a bowl, whisk the eggs with salt and pepper.
2. Heat olive oil in a non-stick skillet over medium heat. Add spinach and sauté until wilted.
3. Pour the eggs over the spinach and cook until the edges start to set.
4. Sprinkle feta cheese on top, fold the omelet, and cook for another minute.
5. Serve warm.

QUINOA SALAD WITH CHICKPEAS AND VEGGIES

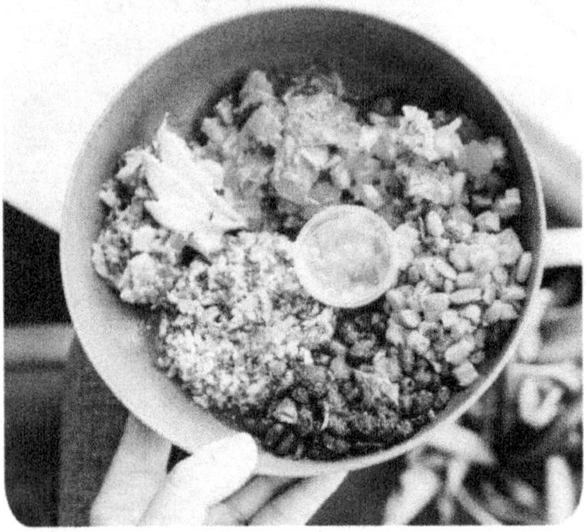

1 bowl

MACROS

- Calories: 350
- Protein: 12g
- Carbohydrates: 50g
- Fat: 14g

INGREDIENTS

- 1 cup cooked quinoa
- 1/2 cup canned chickpeas, rinsed and drained
- 1/2 cup diced cucumber
- 1/2 cup cherry tomatoes, halved
- 1/4 cup red onion, diced
- 2 tablespoons olive oil
- Juice of 1 lemon
- Salt and pepper to taste
- Fresh parsley for garnish

DIRECTIONS

1. In a large bowl, combine cooked quinoa, chickpeas, cucumber, cherry tomatoes, and red onion.
2. In a small bowl, whisk together olive oil, lemon juice, salt, and pepper.
3. Pour the dressing over the salad and toss to combine.
4. Garnish with fresh parsley and serve chilled or at room temperature.

TURKEY AND AVOCADO WRAP

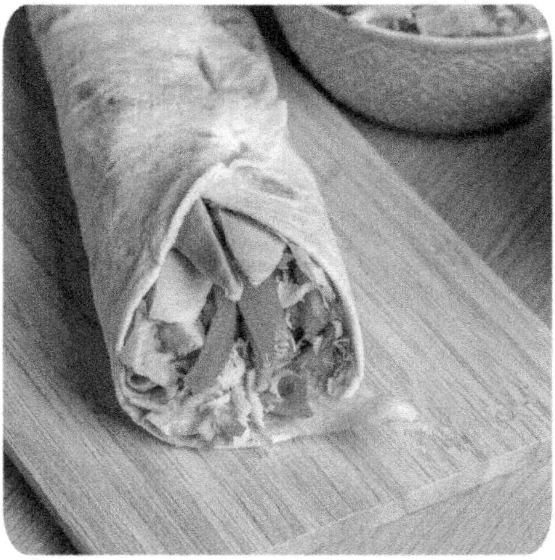

1 wrap

MACROS

- Calories: 350
- Protein: 25g
- Carbohydrates: 30g
- Fat: 15g

INGREDIENTS

- 1 whole grain wrap or tortilla
- 4 oz sliced turkey breast
- 1/2 avocado, sliced
- 1/2 cup mixed greens
- 1/4 cup sliced bell peppers
- Mustard or hummus for spreading

DIRECTIONS

1. Spread mustard or hummus on the wrap.
2. Layer turkey, avocado, mixed greens, and bell peppers on top.
3. Roll the wrap tightly and slice in half.
4. Enjoy with a side of fresh fruit or veggie sticks.

BAKED SALMON WITH ROASTED VEGETABLES

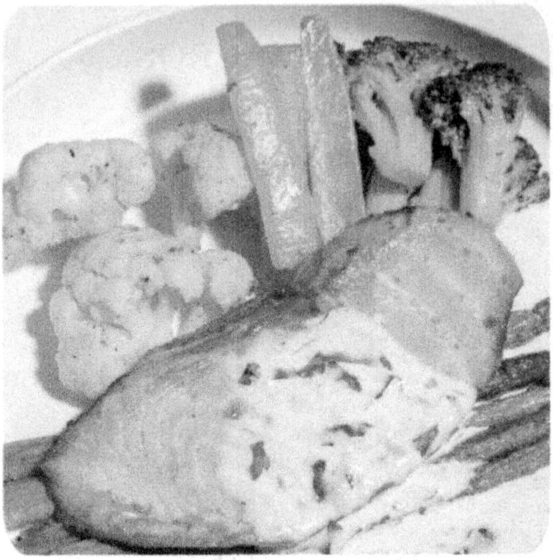

1 fillet with vegetables

MACROS

- Calories: 350
- Protein: 30g
- Carbohydrates: 15g
- Fat: 20g

INGREDIENTS

- 2 salmon fillets
- 1 cup broccoli florets
- 1 cup cauliflower florets
- 1 tablespoon olive oil
- 1 teaspoon garlic powder
- Salt and pepper to taste
- Lemon wedges for serving

DIRECTIONS

1. Preheat the oven to 400°F (200°C).
2. On a baking sheet, toss broccoli and cauliflower with olive oil, garlic powder, salt, and pepper.
3. Place salmon fillets on the baking sheet and season with salt and pepper.
4. Bake for 15-20 minutes, or until the salmon is cooked through and vegetables are tender.
5. Serve with lemon wedges.

LENTIL AND VEGETABLE STIR-FRY

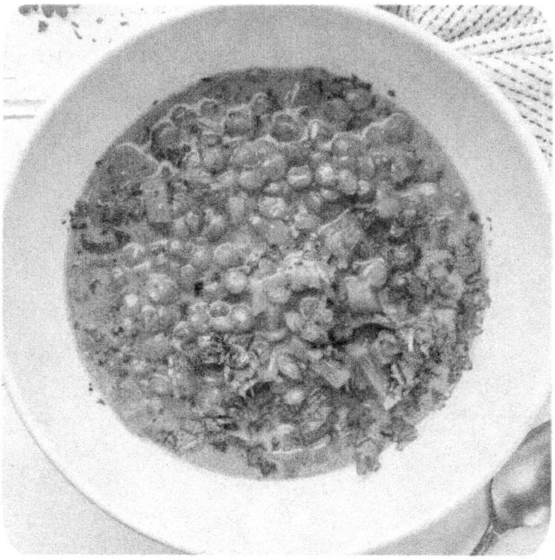

1 bowl

MACROS

- Calories: 400
- Protein: 20g
- Carbohydrates: 60g
- Fat: 10g

INGREDIENTS

- 1 cup cooked lentils
- 1 cup mixed vegetables (bell peppers, carrots, snap peas)
- 2 tablespoons soy sauce (or tamari for gluten-free)
- 1 tablespoon sesame oil
- 1 teaspoon ginger, minced
- 1 teaspoon garlic, minced
- Cooked brown rice or quinoa for serving

DIRECTIONS

1. In a large skillet, heat sesame oil over medium heat. Add ginger and garlic, and sauté for 1 minute.
2. Add mixed vegetables and stir-fry until tender.
3. Stir in cooked lentils and soy sauce, cooking until heated through.
4. Serve over brown rice or quinoa.

HUMMUS AND VEGGIE STICKS

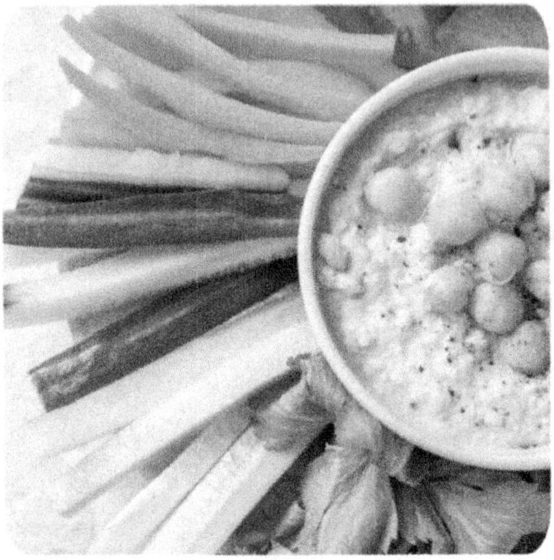

1/2 cup hummus with assorted veggies

MACROS

- Calories: 200
- Protein: 6g
- Carbohydrates: 20g
- Fat: 10g

INGREDIENTS

- 1 cup hummus (store-bought or homemade)
- Assorted veggie sticks (carrots, celery, cucumber, bell peppers)

DIRECTIONS

1. Arrange veggie sticks on a plate.
2. Serve with hummus for dipping.

GREEK YOGURT PARFAIT

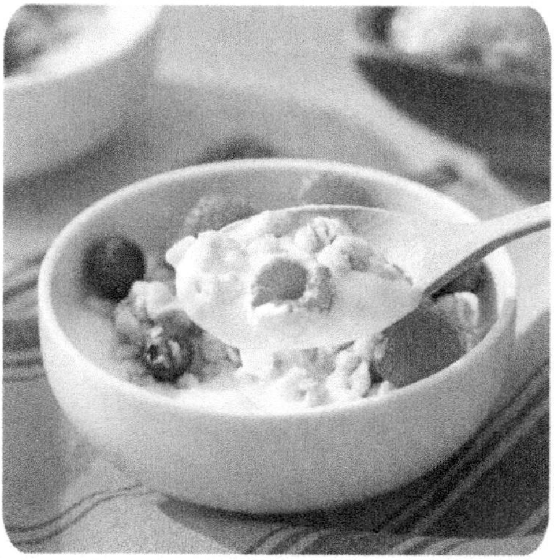

1 Parfait

MACROS

- Calories: 250
- Protein: 20g
- Carbohydrates: 30g
- Fat: 5g

INGREDIENTS

- 1 cup plain Greek yogurt
- 1/2 cup mixed berries
- 1 tablespoon honey (optional)
- 2 tablespoons granola or nuts

DIRECTIONS

1. In a glass or bowl, layer Greek yogurt, mixed berries, and honey.
2. Top with granola or nuts for added crunch.
3. Enjoy as a satisfying snack or light dessert.

Chapter 6: Meal Planning Made Simple

Meal planning is a powerful tool for managing PCOS and supporting your health goals. By organizing your meals in advance, you can ensure that you're making nutritious choices that align with your dietary needs. This chapter will guide you through creating a weekly meal plan, provide tips for batch cooking and meal prep, and offer sample meal plans for different dietary preferences.

How to Create a Weekly Meal Plan

Step 1: Assess Your Schedule

- Take a look at your week ahead and identify busy days when you may need quick meals or snacks.
- Consider any social events or dining out that may affect your meal planning.

Step 2: Choose Your Meals

- Select recipes that incorporate the foods from the PCOS food list. Aim for a balance of protein, healthy fats, and complex carbohydrates.
- Include a variety of fruits and vegetables to ensure you're getting a wide range of nutrients.

Step 3: Create a Shopping List

- Based on your chosen recipes, compile a shopping list of ingredients you'll need for the week.
- Organize your list by food categories (fruits, vegetables, proteins, grains, etc.) to make shopping easier.

Step 4: Prepare Your Meals

- Set aside time for meal prep, ideally on a day when you have a few hours to dedicate to cooking.
- Cook larger batches of grains, proteins, and roasted vegetables that can be used in multiple meals throughout the week.

Step 5: Store and Label

- Use clear containers to store your meals and snacks. Label them with the contents and date to keep track of freshness.

- Consider portion sizes to help with meal control and to make it easier to grab meals on busy days.

Tips for Batch Cooking and Meal Prep

- Plan for Leftovers: Cook larger portions of meals that can be easily reheated for lunch or dinner the next day.
- Use Versatile Ingredients: Choose ingredients that can be used in multiple recipes, such as quinoa, chicken, or roasted vegetables.
- Invest in Quality Containers: Use glass or BPA-free plastic containers that are microwave and dishwasher safe for easy storage and reheating.
- Prep Snacks in Advance: Cut up veggies, portion out hummus, or prepare fruit cups for quick, healthy snacks throughout the week.
- Make Freezer-Friendly Meals: Prepare meals that can be frozen and reheated later, such as soups, stews, or casseroles.

Sample Meal Plans for Different Dietary Preferences

Sample Meal Plan: Omnivore

Day 1

- Breakfast: Berry Smoothie Bowl
    - Macros: 300 calories, 5g protein, 50g carbs, 10g fat
- Lunch: Quinoa Salad with Chickpeas and Veggies
    - Macros: 350 calories, 12g protein, 50g carbs, 14g fat
- Dinner: Baked Salmon with Roasted Vegetables
    - Macros: 350 calories, 30g protein, 15g carbs, 20g fat
- Snack: Hummus and Veggie Sticks
    - Macros: 200 calories, 6g protein, 20g carbs, 10g fat

Total Daily Macros:

1200 calories, 53g protein, 135g carbs, 54g fat

Sample Meal Plan: Vegetarian

Day 1

- Breakfast: Spinach and Feta Omelet
    - Macros: 200 calories, 14g protein, 2g carbs, 15g fat
- Lunch: Lentil and Vegetable Stir-Fry
    - Macros: 400 calories, 20g protein, 60g carbs, 10g fat

- Dinner: Stuffed Bell Peppers (with quinoa, black beans, and veggies)
    - Macros: 350 calories, 15g protein, 50g carbs, 10g fat
- Snack: Greek Yogurt Parfait
    - Macros: 250 calories, 20g protein, 30g carbs, 5g fat

Total Daily Macros:

1200 calories, 69g protein, 142g carbs, 40g fat

Sample Meal Plan: Vegan

Day 1

- Breakfast: Chia Seed Pudding (made with almond milk and topped with berries)
    - Macros: 250 calories, 8g protein, 30g carbs, 12g fat
- Lunch: Quinoa and Black Bean Bowl (with avocado and salsa)
    - Macros: 400 calories, 15g protein, 60g carbs, 10g fat
- Dinner: Vegetable Stir-Fry with Tofu
    - Macros: 350 calories, 20g protein, 40g carbs, 15g fat
- Snack: Apple with Almond Butter
    - Macros: 200 calories, 4g protein, 25g carbs, 10g fat

Total Daily Macros:

1200 calories, 47g protein, 155g carbs, 47g fat

These sample meal plans provide a framework for incorporating PCOS-friendly foods into your diet while accommodating different dietary preferences. Adjust portion sizes and ingredients as needed to meet your individual nutritional needs and preferences.

Chapter 7: Navigating Social Situations

Managing PCOS and making healthy dietary choices can be challenging, especially in social situations. Whether you're dining out, attending family gatherings, or celebrating holidays, having a plan can help you stay on track with your health goals. This chapter provides practical tips for making healthy choices in various social settings.

Tips for Eating Out: Making Healthy Choices at Restaurants

- ***Review the Menu in Advance***: Many restaurants have their menus available online. Take a look before you go to identify healthier options that align with your dietary needs.

- ***Choose Whole Foods***: Opt for dishes that feature whole, minimally processed ingredients. Look for items that include plenty of vegetables, lean proteins, and whole grains.
- ***Watch Portion Sizes***: Restaurant portions can be larger than what you would typically serve at home. Consider sharing a dish with a friend or asking for a half portion if available.
- ***Ask for Modifications***: Don't hesitate to request modifications to your meal. Ask for dressings and sauces on the side, substitute fried items for grilled or steamed options, and request whole grain alternatives when possible.
- ***Be Mindful of Beverages***: Choose water, herbal tea, or unsweetened beverages instead of sugary drinks or high-calorie cocktails. If you choose to drink alcohol, opt for lower-calorie options like wine or spirits mixed with soda water.
- ***Listen to Your Body***: Pay attention to your hunger and fullness cues. Eat slowly and savor your meal, allowing your body to signal when it's satisfied.

How to Handle Holidays and Family Gatherings

- ***Plan Ahead***: If you know you'll be attending a holiday gathering, plan your meals for the day accordingly. Consider eating a healthy snack before the event to avoid arriving overly hungry.
- ***Bring a Dish***: Offer to bring a healthy dish to share. This ensures there will be at least one option that aligns with your dietary preferences. Consider making a colorful

salad, a vegetable platter with hummus, or a healthy dessert.

- ***Focus on the Company***: Remember that holidays and gatherings are about spending time with loved ones. Engage in conversations and activities rather than solely focusing on food.
- ***Practice Moderation***: It's okay to enjoy traditional holiday foods in moderation. Allow yourself to indulge in small portions of your favorite dishes while prioritizing healthier options.
- ***Stay Active***: Incorporate physical activity into your holiday plans. Consider going for a walk with family after a meal or participating in fun activities that keep you moving.

Strategies for Communicating Your Dietary Needs

- ***Be Open and Honest***: When discussing your dietary needs with friends and family, be open about your health goals and the reasons behind your choices. Most people will be supportive and understanding.
- ***Use "I" Statements***: Frame your dietary needs in a positive way. For example, say, "I'm focusing on eating more whole foods to support my health," rather than "I can't eat that."
- ***Educate Others***: If appropriate, share information about PCOS and how certain foods affect your health. This can help others understand your choices and may encourage them to make healthier choices as well.
- ***Offer Alternatives***: If you're attending a gathering where food is served, suggest alternatives that align with your dietary needs. For example, if dessert is being served, offer to bring a healthier option that everyone can enjoy.

- ***Practice Self-Compassion***: Remember that it's okay to have moments of indulgence. If you find yourself in a situation where you eat something that doesn't align with your goals, don't be too hard on yourself. Focus on getting back on track with your next meal.

Navigating social situations while managing PCOS can be challenging, but with the right strategies and mindset, you can enjoy your time with friends and family while making choices that support your health.

Chapter 8: Mindset Matters

The journey to conception can be filled with ups and downs, especially for women managing Polycystic Ovary Syndrome (PCOS). While dietary and lifestyle changes are crucial, cultivating a positive mindset is equally important. This chapter explores the significance of a positive mindset in your TTC journey and offers journaling prompts and exercises to support your emotional well-being.

The Importance of a Positive Mindset in Your TTC Journey

- ***Reduces Stress and Anxiety***: A positive mindset can help alleviate the stress and anxiety that often accompany the TTC journey. Stress can negatively impact hormonal balance and fertility, making it essential to find ways to manage it effectively.

- ***Enhances Resilience***: Maintaining a positive outlook can foster resilience, allowing you to navigate challenges with greater ease. When faced with setbacks, a positive mindset helps you bounce back and stay focused on your goals.
- ***Promotes Self-Compassion***: A positive mindset encourages self-compassion, allowing you to treat yourself with kindness and understanding. This is especially important during times of frustration or disappointment, as it helps you maintain a healthy relationship with yourself.
- ***Encourages Healthy Choices***: When you approach your TTC journey with a positive mindset, you're more likely to make choices that support your health and well-being. This includes sticking to your dietary goals, engaging in regular physical activity, and prioritizing self-care.
- ***Fosters a Supportive Community***: A positive mindset can attract supportive relationships and communities. Surrounding yourself with like-minded individuals who share your goals can provide encouragement and motivation throughout your journey.

Journaling Prompts and Exercises for Emotional Well-Being

Journaling Prompts

- ***Gratitude List***: Write down three things you are grateful for each day. This practice can help shift your focus from challenges to the positive aspects of your life.
- ***Affirmations***: Create a list of positive affirmations related to your TTC journey. For example, "I am taking

steps to support my health and fertility" or "I trust my body's ability to conceive." Repeat these affirmations daily.

- ***Reflect on Your Journey***: Take time to reflect on your TTC journey. Write about your feelings, experiences, and any lessons learned. Acknowledge both the highs and lows, and celebrate your progress.
- ***Visualize Your Goals***: Write a detailed description of your vision for the future. What does your life look like when you achieve your TTC goals? Include emotions, experiences, and the environment you envision.
- ***Identify Fears and Concerns***: Write about any fears or concerns you have regarding your TTC journey. Acknowledge these feelings and consider how you can address or reframe them positively.

Exercises for Emotional Well-Being

- ***Mindfulness Meditation***: Set aside a few minutes each day for mindfulness meditation. Focus on your breath and allow yourself to be present in the moment. This practice can help reduce stress and promote emotional clarity.
- ***Gratitude Journaling***: Dedicate a journal specifically for gratitude. Each day, write down three things you appreciate about yourself, your journey, or your support system. This exercise can help cultivate a positive mindset.
- ***Vision Board***: Create a vision board that represents your goals and aspirations related to your TTC journey. Include images, quotes, and words that inspire you. Place it somewhere visible to remind you of your intentions.
- ***Positive Self-Talk***: Pay attention to your inner dialogue. Challenge negative thoughts and replace them with positive affirmations. For example, if you catch

yourself thinking, "I'll never conceive," reframe it to, "I am taking steps to support my fertility."

- ***Connect with Supportive Communities***: Seek out online or local support groups for women with PCOS or those on a TTC journey. Sharing experiences and connecting with others can provide encouragement and a sense of belonging.

By prioritizing a positive mindset and engaging in these journaling prompts and exercises, you can enhance your emotional well-being and navigate your TTC journey with greater confidence and resilience.

Chapter 9: Supplements and Nutritional Support

While a balanced diet is the foundation of good health, certain supplements can provide additional nutritional support for women with Polycystic Ovary Syndrome (PCOS) who are trying to conceive. This chapter explores various supplements that may support fertility, their benefits, recommended dosages, and guidance on how to choose quality products.

Overview of Supplements that May Support Fertility

1. Inositol

- **What It Is**: Inositol is a carbohydrate that plays a role in insulin signaling and hormone regulation.
- **Benefits:**
    - Improves insulin sensitivity, which is crucial for managing PCOS.
    - Regulates menstrual cycles and enhances ovarian function.
    - May improve egg quality and fertility outcomes.
- **Recommended Dosage**: 2,000 to 4,000 mg per day, typically taken in two divided doses (morning and evening).
- **When to Take**: It can be taken with or without food, but consistency is key for optimal results.

2. Folic Acid

- **What It Is:** Folic acid is a B-vitamin essential for DNA synthesis and cell division.
- **Benefits**:
    - Crucial for women trying to conceive, as it helps prevent neural tube defects in the developing fetus.
    - Supports overall reproductive health and may improve fertility.
- **Recommended Dosage**: 400 to 800 mcg per day, starting at least one month before conception and continuing through the first trimester of pregnancy.

- **When to Take**: It can be taken at any time of day, with or without food.

3. Vitamin D

- **What It Is**: Vitamin D is a fat-soluble vitamin that plays a role in calcium metabolism and immune function.
- **Benefits**:
    - Adequate vitamin D levels may improve insulin sensitivity and reproductive health in women with PCOS.
    - Supports ovarian function and may enhance fertility.
- **Recommended Dosage**: 1,000 to 2,000 IU per day, depending on individual needs and blood levels.
- **When to Take**: Best taken with a meal that contains fat to enhance absorption.

4. Omega-3 Fatty Acids

- **What It Is**: Omega-3 fatty acids are essential fats found in fish oil and certain plant sources.
- **Benefits:**
    - Have anti-inflammatory properties that may help improve insulin sensitivity and support overall reproductive health.
    - May promote a healthy pregnancy and improve egg quality.
- **Recommended Dosage**: 1,000 to 2,000 mg of combined EPA and DHA (the two main types of omega-3s) per day.
- **When to Take**: Can be taken with meals to reduce the risk of gastrointestinal discomfort.

5. Coenzyme Q10 (CoQ10)

- **What It Is**: CoQ10 is a powerful antioxidant that helps produce energy in cells.
- **Benefits**:
    - May improve egg quality and ovarian function, particularly in women with diminished ovarian reserve.
    - Supports overall cellular health and energy production.
- **Recommended Dosage**: 100 to 300 mg per day, divided into two doses.
- **When to Take**: Best taken with meals to enhance absorption.

6. Zinc

- **What It Is:** Zinc is a trace mineral that plays a role in numerous biological processes, including immune function and hormone regulation.
- **Benefits**:
    - Adequate zinc levels are important for reproductive health and may help improve fertility in women with PCOS.
    - Supports hormone balance and immune function.
- **Recommended Dosage**: 15 to 30 mg per day.
- **When to Take**: Can be taken with or without food, but taking it with food may help reduce stomach upset.

7. Magnesium

- **What It Is:** Magnesium is a mineral involved in over 300 biochemical reactions in the body.

- **Benefits:**
    - May help regulate blood sugar levels and improve insulin sensitivity, making it beneficial for women with PCOS.
    - Supports overall hormonal balance and can help alleviate symptoms of PMS.
- **Recommended Dosage**: 300 to 400 mg per day.
- **When to Take**: Best taken in the evening, as it may promote relaxation and improve sleep quality.

How to Choose Quality Supplements

- ***Look for Third-Party Testing***: Choose supplements that have been tested by independent organizations for quality and purity. Look for seals from organizations like NSF International or US Pharmacopeia (USP).
- ***Check the Ingredients***: Review the ingredient list for any fillers, artificial colors, or preservatives. Opt for supplements with minimal ingredients and those that are free from allergens.
- ***Consider Bioavailability***: Some forms of vitamins and minerals are better absorbed by the body than others. For example, choose methylated forms of B vitamins or chelated minerals for better absorption.
- ***Consult with a Healthcare Professional***: Before starting any new supplement regimen, consult with a healthcare provider or a registered dietitian. They can help assess your individual needs and recommend appropriate supplements based on your health status and goals.
- ***Read Reviews and Research***: Look for reputable brands with positive reviews and a history of quality.

Research the company's reputation and commitment to quality control.

- ***Be Mindful of Dosages***: Follow the recommended dosages on the supplement label or as advised by your healthcare provider. More is not always better, and excessive intake of certain vitamins and minerals can be harmful.

By incorporating the right supplements into your routine and choosing high-quality products, you can provide additional nutritional support for your fertility journey. Remember that supplements should complement a balanced diet, not replace it.

Chapter 10: Tracking Your Progress

Monitoring your progress is an essential part of managing Polycystic Ovary Syndrome (PCOS) and supporting your fertility journey. By keeping track of your symptoms, dietary changes, and overall health, you can gain valuable insights into what works best for your body. This chapter provides guidance on how to effectively monitor your progress and introduces tools and apps that can assist you in this process.

How to Monitor Your Symptoms and Dietary Changes

1. Keep a Symptom Journal

What to Track: Record your daily symptoms, including menstrual cycle changes, mood fluctuations, energy levels, and any physical symptoms such as acne or weight changes.

How to Use It:

- *Choose a Format*: Use a physical notebook, a digital document, or a dedicated app to log your symptoms daily.
- *Be Consistent*: Set a specific time each day to fill out your journal, such as in the morning or before bed.
- *Include Details*: Note the severity of symptoms on a scale (e.g., 1-10) and any potential triggers (e.g., stress, certain foods).
- *Review Regularly:* At the end of each week or month, review your entries to identify patterns or changes in your symptoms.

2. Food Diary

What to Track: Write down everything you eat and drink, including portion sizes and any snacks. Note how you feel after meals, including energy levels and cravings.

How to Use It:

- *Select a Method*: Use a notebook, a food tracking app, or a spreadsheet to log your meals.
- *Be Detailed*: Include specific ingredients, cooking methods, and portion sizes to get an accurate picture of your intake.

- *Reflect on Feelings*: After each meal, jot down how you felt physically and emotionally. Did you experience any cravings or energy dips?
- *Analyze Trends*: After a week, look for correlations between your food choices and how you felt. This can help you identify foods that support your well-being.

3. Monitor Your Menstrual Cycle

What to Track: Keep track of your menstrual cycle length, flow, and any associated symptoms. Note any irregularities or changes in your cycle.

How to Use It:

- *Choose a Tracking Method*: Use a calendar, a cycle tracking app, or a journal to log your cycle details.
- *Record Key Dates*: Mark the first day of your period, the length of your cycle, and any symptoms experienced (e.g., cramps, mood changes).
- *Look for Patterns*: Over time, analyze your cycle data to identify any irregularities or trends, such as changes in cycle length or symptoms.

4. Set Specific Goals

What to Track: Establish clear, achievable goals related to your diet, exercise, and symptom management.

How to Use It:

- *Write Down Your Goals*: Be specific about what you want to achieve (e.g., "I will eat at least 5 servings of vegetables each day").
- *Break It Down*: Divide larger goals into smaller, manageable steps to make them more achievable.

- *Track Progress*: Use a checklist or app to monitor your progress toward your goals. Celebrate small victories along the way.

5. Regular Check-Ins

What to Track: Schedule regular check-ins with yourself to review your progress.

How to Use It:

- *Set a Schedule*: Choose a specific day and time each week or month for your check-in.
- *Reflect on Your Journey*: Review your symptom journal, food diary, and goals. Consider what's working and what challenges you're facing.
- *Adjust as Needed*: Based on your reflections, make any necessary adjustments to your diet, lifestyle, or goals.

Tools and Apps for Tracking Food Intake and Cycle Changes

1. MyFitnessPal

- Overview: A popular app for tracking food intake, exercise, and weight loss. It has a large database of foods and allows you to log meals easily.
- How to Use: Create an account, set your dietary goals, and start logging your meals. Use the barcode scanner for quick entry.

2. Clue

- Overview: A menstrual cycle tracking app that helps you monitor your cycle, symptoms, and fertility windows.

- How to Use: Input your cycle data, including start and end dates, flow, and symptoms. The app will provide insights and predictions based on your data.

3. Ovia Fertility

- Overview: An app designed for women trying to conceive, offering cycle tracking, symptom logging, and personalized insights.
- How to Use: Log your cycle details, symptoms, and any fertility-related information. The app will help you identify patterns and provide fertility predictions.

4. Cronometer

- Overview: A comprehensive nutrition tracking app that provides detailed information on micronutrients and macronutrients.
- How to Use: Create an account, set your dietary goals, and log your food intake. The app will provide detailed nutrient breakdowns.

5. Fitbit

- Overview: A fitness tracker that monitors physical activity, sleep patterns, and heart rate. The accompanying app allows for food logging and goal setting.
- How to Use: Sync your Fitbit device with the app, log your meals, and track your activity levels. Set fitness goals and monitor your progress.

6. Google Sheets or Excel

- Overview: For those who prefer a more manual approach, using a spreadsheet can be an effective way to track food intake, symptoms, and cycle changes.
- How to Use: Create a custom template to log your data. Use formulas to calculate totals and create graphs for visual progress tracking.

By actively tracking your symptoms, dietary changes, and overall health, you can gain valuable insights into your body's responses and make informed decisions that support your PCOS management and fertility journey. Utilizing tools and apps can simplify this process and help you stay organized and motivated.

Chapter 11: Success Stories and Testimonials

Managing Polycystic Ovary Syndrome (PCOS) can be a challenging journey, but many women have found success through dietary changes and lifestyle adjustments. In this chapter, we share inspirational stories from women who have successfully managed their PCOS symptoms through nutrition, along with valuable tips and advice for those on a similar path.

Inspirational Stories

Sarah's Journey to Balance

Sarah, a 32-year-old teacher, struggled with irregular periods, weight gain, and fatigue for years after her PCOS diagnosis.

Frustrated with her symptoms, she decided to take control of her health.

Sarah began by eliminating processed foods and focusing on whole, nutrient-dense options. She incorporated more fruits, vegetables, lean proteins, and healthy fats into her meals. She also started tracking her food intake to better understand her eating habits.

Within a few months, Sarah noticed significant improvements. Her menstrual cycles became more regular, and she lost 15 pounds. She felt more energetic and was able to engage in physical activities she once found challenging.

"Start small and be patient with yourself. Celebrate every little victory, and don't be afraid to ask for support from friends and family. You're not alone in this journey!"

Emily's Transformation

Emily, a 28-year-old graphic designer, faced challenges with acne, weight gain, and mood swings due to PCOS. After feeling overwhelmed, she sought help from a nutritionist.

With guidance, Emily adopted a low-glycemic diet, focusing on whole grains, legumes, and plenty of vegetables. She also began meal prepping to ensure she had healthy options readily available.

After six months, Emily experienced clearer skin, improved mood stability, and a 20-pound weight loss. She felt empowered by her ability to manage her symptoms through nutrition.

"Don't be afraid to seek help from professionals. A nutritionist helped me understand how food affects my body, and it made all the difference. Also, find a community of women who understand what you're going through."

Jessica's Holistic Approach

Jessica, a 35-year-old mother of two, was diagnosed with PCOS after struggling with infertility. Determined to conceive, she focused on improving her overall health.

Jessica embraced a holistic approach, incorporating not only dietary changes but also mindfulness practices. She eliminated refined sugars and processed foods, focusing on a balanced diet rich in whole foods. She also practiced yoga and meditation to reduce stress.

After a year of commitment to her health, Jessica successfully conceived and gave birth to a healthy baby. She continues to prioritize nutrition and self-care in her daily life.

"It's not just about food; it's about your overall well-being. Incorporate stress-reducing practices into your routine, and don't hesitate to explore different avenues for support. Your journey is unique, and it's okay to take your time."

Tips and Advice from Those Who Have Been on the Journey

- Stay Informed: Educate yourself about PCOS and how nutrition impacts your symptoms. Knowledge is empowering and can help you make informed choices.
- Set Realistic Goals: Focus on small, achievable goals rather than drastic changes. Celebrate your progress, no matter how small.
- Find Support: Connect with others who understand your journey. Online forums, support groups, or local meetups can provide encouragement and motivation.
- Be Kind to Yourself: Understand that managing PCOS is a journey with ups and downs. Practice self-compassion and avoid negative self-talk.
- Experiment with Foods: Everyone's body is different. Pay attention to how certain foods make you feel and adjust your diet accordingly. Don't be afraid to try new recipes and ingredients.
- Prioritize Self-Care: Make time for activities that bring you joy and relaxation. Whether it's reading, exercising, or spending time with loved ones, self-care is essential for emotional well-being.
- Consult Professionals: Seek guidance from healthcare providers, nutritionists, or dietitians who specialize in PCOS. They can provide personalized advice and support tailored to your needs.

These success stories and tips serve as a reminder that with dedication, support, and the right approach, it is possible to manage PCOS effectively and improve your quality of life. Remember, you are not alone on this journey, and there is hope for a healthier future.

Chapter 12: Conclusion and Next Steps

As you reach the end of this book, it's important to reflect on the journey you've undertaken and the knowledge you've gained about managing Polycystic Ovary Syndrome (PCOS) through nutrition and lifestyle changes. This chapter recaps the key takeaways, offers encouragement for the journey ahead, and provides resources for further reading and support.

Recap of Key Takeaways

- Understanding PCOS: Recognizing the symptoms and challenges associated with PCOS is the first step toward effective management. Knowledge empowers you to make informed decisions about your health.

- Nutrition Matters: A balanced diet rich in whole foods, healthy fats, lean proteins, and low-glycemic carbohydrates can significantly impact your symptoms and overall well-being. Incorporating fertility-boosting foods can enhance your chances of conception.
- Mindset is Key: Cultivating a positive mindset is essential for navigating the ups and downs of the TTC journey. Practicing self-compassion, gratitude, and mindfulness can help you stay focused and resilient.
- Tracking Progress: Monitoring your symptoms, dietary changes, and menstrual cycles can provide valuable insights into your health. Utilizing tools and apps can simplify this process and help you stay organized.
- Support is Available: Connecting with healthcare professionals, support groups, and online communities can provide encouragement and guidance. You don't have to navigate this journey alone.
- Supplements for Support: Certain supplements, such as inositol, folic acid, and omega-3 fatty acids, can provide additional nutritional support for managing PCOS and enhancing fertility. Always consult with a healthcare provider before starting any new supplements.

Encouragement for the Journey Ahead

As you continue on your journey to manage PCOS and support your fertility, remember that progress takes time. Be patient with yourself and celebrate the small victories along the way. Each step you take toward better health is a step in the right direction.

It's normal to encounter challenges and setbacks, but don't lose sight of your goals. Surround yourself with supportive individuals who understand your journey, and don't hesitate to seek help when needed. Your health and well-being are worth the effort.

Resources for Further Reading and Support

- Books:
  - "The PCOS Diet Book" by Colette Harris and Theresa Cheung
  - "The Fertility Diet" by Jorge E. Chavarro, Walter C. Willett, and Patrick J. Skerrett
  - "PCOS: The Ultimate Guide to Managing Your PCOS" by Dr. Fiona McCulloch
- Websites:
  - 1: A resource for information, support, and advocacy for women with PCOS.
  - 2: Offers resources and information on reproductive health and fertility.
  - 3: Provides support and resources for individuals facing infertility.
- Support Groups:
  - Look for local or online support groups for women with PCOS. Connecting with others who share similar experiences can provide encouragement and understanding.
- Healthcare Professionals:
  - Consider working with a registered dietitian, nutritionist, or healthcare provider who specializes in PCOS. They can provide personalized guidance and support tailored to your needs.

As you move forward, remember that you have the power to take charge of your health and well-being. Embrace the journey, stay committed to your goals, and know that you are not alone. With the right tools, support, and mindset, you can successfully manage PCOS and enhance your fertility.

A Note of Thanks

Hey Sis,

Thank you for taking the time to read "The No-Diet PCOS Fertility Food List & Meal Plan." I hope that the information, recipes, and strategies shared within these pages have empowered you on your journey to manage PCOS and enhance your fertility.

As a fellow traveler on this path, I understand the challenges and triumphs that come with navigating PCOS. Remember, you are not alone in this journey. Each step you take toward better health is a testament to your strength and resilience. Embrace the process, celebrate your victories—big and small—and be kind to yourself along the way.

I encourage you to continue exploring, learning, and connecting with others who share similar experiences. Your health and well-being are worth the effort, and with the right tools and support, you can achieve your goals.

Thank you for allowing me to be a part of your journey. I wish you all the best as you move forward, and may you find joy, hope, and success in every step you take.

With warmest wishes,

Giselle

We Value Your Feedback!

Thank you for reading "The No-Diet PCOS Fertility Food List & Meal Plan"! Your thoughts and experiences are incredibly important to us, and we would love to hear your feedback.

If you found this book helpful, please consider taking a moment to leave a review on Amazon. Your review not only helps us improve future editions but also assists other readers in finding the support they need on their journey with PCOS.

How to Leave a Review:

- Visit the Amazon page for the book.
- Click on the "Write a Customer Review" button.
- Share your thoughts and experiences!

You can also scan the QR code below to be directed to the review page:

https://go.binnovatedigital.com/PCOSfoodlist

Thank you for your support and for being a part of our community! Together, we can empower more women to manage PCOS and embrace their health journeys.

Resources and References

- Azziz, R., Carmina, E., Chen, Z., et al. (2004). "Polycystic ovary syndrome." *Nature Reviews Disease Primers*, 1, 1-12. 1
- Teede, H. J., Deeks, A. A., & Moran, L. J. (2010). "Polycystic ovary syndrome: a complex condition with psychological, reproductive and metabolic manifestations." *Australian and New Zealand Journal of Obstetrics and Gynaecology*, 50(1), 1-8. 2
- Chiu, T. H., & Chen, C. Y. (2018). "Dietary interventions for women with polycystic ovary syndrome: A systematic review." *Journal of the American College of Nutrition*, 37(5), 421-429. 3
- Dunaif, A. (1997). "Insulin resistance and the polycystic ovary syndrome: mechanisms and implications for pathogenesis." *Endocrine Reviews*, 18(6), 774-800. 1
- Legro, R. S., et al. (2007). "The effect of weight loss on reproductive function in women with polycystic ovary syndrome." *Obstetrics & Gynecology*, 109(2), 309-317. 2
- Palomba, S., et al. (2015). "Polycystic ovary syndrome: a comprehensive review of the role of diet and lifestyle." *Journal of Endocrinological Investigation*, 38(1), 1-12. 3
- Chavarro, J. E., et al. (2007). "Diet and fertility: a review." *American Journal of Clinical Nutrition*, 85(5), 1257-1262. 1
- Gaskins, A. J., & Chavarro, J. E. (2018). "Diet and fertility: a review." *Current Opinion in Obstetrics and Gynecology*, 30(3), 145-151. 2

- Rojas, J. M., et al. (2019). "Dietary patterns and fertility: a systematic review." *Nutrients*, 11(4), 1-20. 3
- Slavin, J. L. (2005). "Why whole grains are protective: biological mechanisms." *Proceedings of the Nutrition Society*, 64(1), 19-24. 1
- Hu, F. B. (2002). "Resistant starch, glycemic index, and the risk of type 2 diabetes." *Diabetes Care*, 25(2), 353-354. 2
- Mozaffarian, D., et al. (2011). "Changes in diet and lifestyle and long-term weight gain in women and men." *New England Journal of Medicine*, 364(25), 2392-2404. 3

Made in the USA
Monee, IL
04 November 2026

67383106R00066